高位骶骨肿瘤外科治疗结局

梁伟明　著

广西科学技术出版社

·南宁·

图书在版编目（CIP）数据

高位骶骨肿瘤外科治疗结局 / 梁伟明著. —南宁：
广西科学技术出版社，2023.9
ISBN 978-7-5551-2056-8

Ⅰ. ①高⋯ Ⅱ. ①梁⋯ Ⅲ. ①骨肿瘤—外科手术
Ⅳ. ①R738.1

中国国家版本馆CIP数据核字（2023）第176808号

高位骶骨肿瘤外科治疗结局

梁伟明　著

责任编辑：李　媛　　　　　　　　　装帧设计：韦宇星
助理编辑：黎　奚　　　　　　　　　责任校对：吴书丽
责任印制：韦文印

出 版 人：梁　志　　　　　　　出版发行：广西科学技术出版社
社　　　址：广西南宁市东葛路 66 号　　邮政编码：530023
网　　　址：http://www.gxkjs.com

印　　　刷：广西雅图盛印务有限公司

开　　　本：787 mm × 1092 mm　　1/16
字　　　数：157 千字　　　　　　　印　　张：8
版　　　次：2023 年 9 月第 1 版　　　印　　次：2023 年 9 月第 1 次印刷
书　　　号：ISBN 978-7-5551-2056-8
定　　　价：58.00 元

本书由广西科技大学博士基金项目

（合同编号：校科博 20Z13）资助出版

序 言

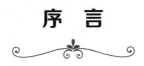

  我曾有幸在北京大学人民医院骨肿瘤科郭卫教授的指导下攻读医学博士学位。读博 3 年期间，我系统地学习了骨肿瘤的相关知识，并参与很多骨肿瘤患者的临床诊治，博士毕业论文的研究内容为高位骶骨恶性肿瘤外科治疗结局，主要包括三个方面：全骶骨切除术后患者的外科治疗结局、健康相关生命质量评价及患者体验的定性分析。毕业至今我就职于广西科技大学第一临床医学院，并对博士期间的研究工作进行了归纳、整理。

  骶骨恶性肿瘤致残率、死亡率高，诊断及治疗的难度很大，其预后效果好坏取决于是否规范化治疗及医生的经验丰富程度。骶骨恶性骨肿瘤患者非常少见，很难在一个医院里积累较多的病例，这对于骨肿瘤临床工作的医生培养造成了一定的困难。本书介绍骶骨部位常见恶性肿瘤的诊治，同时报告一项关于骶骨高位恶性肿瘤外科治疗结局的研究结果：全骶骨切除术后患者的外科治疗结局、健康相关生命质量评价及患者体验的定性分析。本书有助于骨肿瘤相关临床医生了解骶骨恶性肿瘤的预后，对推广骶骨恶性肿瘤的规范化治疗具有积极的作用。

  本书介绍脊索瘤、骨肉瘤、恶性巨细胞瘤、软骨肉瘤、尤因肉瘤、转移瘤等 6 种骶骨部位常见恶性肿瘤的诊治情况，并结合临床研究实际，重点报告全骶骨切除术后患者的外科治疗结局、健康相关生命质量评价及患者体验的定性分析结果，多层面深入了解患者的整体预后，对未来研究高骶骨常见恶性肿瘤进行展望。

  最后，我要特别感谢北京大学人民医院骨肿瘤科郭卫教授及其他老师在我攻读博士学位期间对我的指导和帮助。

梁伟明

2023 年 9 月

目　录

摘　要 ……………………………………………………………………… 1

第1部分　骶骨常见恶性肿瘤的诊治 ……………………………… 4

　1　脊索瘤 ………………………………………………………………… 4

　　1.1　定义 …………………………………………………………………… 4

　　1.2　流行病学 ……………………………………………………………… 4

　　1.3　临床表现 ……………………………………………………………… 4

　　1.4　影像学表现 …………………………………………………………… 5

　　1.5　病理表现 ……………………………………………………………… 5

　　1.6　鉴别诊断 ……………………………………………………………… 5

　　1.7　治疗方法 ……………………………………………………………… 6

　2　恶性骨巨细胞肿瘤 …………………………………………………… 6

　　2.1　定义 …………………………………………………………………… 6

　　2.2　流行病学 ……………………………………………………………… 6

　　2.3　临床表现 ……………………………………………………………… 7

　　2.4　影像学表现 …………………………………………………………… 7

　　2.5　病理表现 ……………………………………………………………… 7

　　2.6　鉴别诊断与分型 ……………………………………………………… 7

　　2.7　治疗方法 ……………………………………………………………… 8

　3　骨肉瘤 ………………………………………………………………… 8

　　3.1　定义 …………………………………………………………………… 8

　　3.2　流行病学 ……………………………………………………………… 9

3.3　临床表现 ·· 9

3.4　影像学表现 ··· 10

3.5　活检 ·· 11

3.6　病理表现 ·· 11

3.7　鉴别诊断 ·· 13

3.8　治疗方法 ·· 13

3.9　预后情况 ·· 14

4　软骨肉瘤 ·· 15

4.1　定义 ·· 15

4.2　流行病学 ·· 15

4.3　临床表现 ·· 15

4.4　影像学表现 ··· 15

4.5　病理表现 ·· 16

4.6　诊断与鉴别诊断 ······································ 18

4.7　治疗方法 ·· 20

5　尤因肉瘤 ·· 23

5.1　定义 ·· 23

5.2　流行病学 ·· 23

5.3　临床表现 ·· 23

5.4　影像学表现 ··· 24

5.5　病理表现 ·· 24

5.6　基因学 ··· 25

5.7　外周循环中尤因肉瘤细胞的分子探测 ········· 25

5.8　诊断与鉴别诊断 ······································ 26

5.9　治疗方法 ·· 27

6　骨转移瘤 ·· 29

6.1　定义及流行病学 ······································· 29

6.2　骨转移瘤致溶骨性破坏的分子基础 ……………………………… 29

6.3　临床表现 ………………………………………………………… 30

6.4　诊断 ……………………………………………………………… 30

6.5　治疗 ……………………………………………………………… 31

第 2 部分　高位骶骨恶性肿瘤外科治疗结局研究 ………35

1　研究背景与意义 ……………………………………………………… 35

1.1　全骶骨切除术治疗高位骶骨恶性肿瘤 ………………………… 35

1.2　全骶骨切除术后患者的神经功能评估 ………………………… 36

1.3　全骶骨切除术后患者的健康相关生命质量 …………………… 38

1.4　全骶骨切除术后患者的生活和情感体验 ……………………… 40

2　研究目的与意义 ……………………………………………………… 41

2.1　研究目的 ………………………………………………………… 41

2.2　研究背景及意义 ………………………………………………… 41

2.3　研究方法 ………………………………………………………… 42

3　全骶骨切除术后患者的外科治疗结局及健康相关生命质量 ……42

3.1　前言 ……………………………………………………………… 42

3.2　研究对象及研究方法 …………………………………………… 43

3.3　研究结果 ………………………………………………………… 49

3.4　讨论 ……………………………………………………………… 57

4　全骶骨切除术后患者体验的定性分析 ……………………………… 62

4.1　前言 ……………………………………………………………… 62

4.2　研究对象和研究方法 …………………………………………… 63

4.3　研究结果 ………………………………………………………… 63

4.4　讨论 ……………………………………………………………… 69

第 3 部分　结论和展望 ·································· 71

1　主要结论 ····································· 71

2　创新点 ······································· 71

3　局限性 ······································· 72

参考文献 ··· 73

附录 1　全骶骨切除术后患者的健康相关生命质量调查问卷 ······ 84

附录 2　论文范例 ··································· 89

摘 要

研究背景

全骶骨切除术是治疗高位骶骨恶性肿瘤的主要方法。已有文献报道全骶骨切除术后的手术并发症、神经功能损伤、肿瘤学预后，但罕有文献报道患者的健康相关生命质量，甚至还没有对患者体验进行定性分析的文献报道。

研究目的

统计全骶骨切除术后患者的肿瘤学预后、手术并发症，评估患者的神经功能结局、健康相关生命质量，探讨健康相关生命质量的影响因素，并分析患者的生活和情感体验，多层面深入了解患者的整体预后，以便临床工作者更好地做出手术决策、管理患者预期及促进患者康复。

研究对象及方法

2007年9月至2017年9月期间，共有52例患者曾于北京人民医院骨与软组织肿瘤中心（简称本中心）行全骶骨切除术，其中失访11例，剩下的41例患者中死亡8例，存活的33例患者均愿意参与本研究；男性18例、女性15例，平均年龄47.4岁；脊索瘤21例，软骨肉瘤5例，骨肉瘤3例，尤因肉瘤2例，神经鞘瘤1例，结肠癌1例。通过电子病历查阅患者围手术期的相关信息，包括患者的手术出血量、手术并发症等信息；通过电话随访了解患者的肿瘤学预后、下肢功能及大小便功能，并使用骶骨切除术后神经功能评分系统评估患者的神经功能结局；通过SF-36 v2量表评估患者的健康相关生命质量，使用统计学方法探讨患者健康相关生命质量的影响因素，使用半结构化访谈的方式对患者体验进行定性分析，平均访谈时间26分钟（范围17～63分钟），访谈主题包括：①日常生活能力；②社会交际情况；③学习或工作情况；④对家庭的影响；⑤对造瘘手术的接受程度；⑥对远期康复指导的需求；⑦对住院期间医疗服务的满意度；⑧对治疗结局的满意度。

研究结果

（1）随访时间为平均 25 个月（范围 4 ～ 93 个月），除去失访患者，41 例患者中复发 13 例，其中死亡 8 例，均死于肿瘤的复发与转移。术中出血量平均值 2771 mL（范围 800 ～ 9000 mL）。出现伤口并发症 14 例，内固定失败 7 例，脑脊液漏 6 例，肠道损伤 2 例。

（2）无复发组患者神经功能结局各项评分的均值和标准差为：下肢运动 1.57 ± 0.88 分，疼痛 1.21 ± 0.57 分，会阴感觉 1.08 ± 0.69 分，排尿困难 1.43 ± 0.88 分，尿失禁 1.29 ± 0.71 分，膀胱感觉 1.07 ± 0.90 分，便秘 1.29 ± 0.76 分，大便失禁 1.68 ± 0.72 分，直肠感觉 1.04 ± 0.74 分，神经功能总分 11.66 ± 4.65 分。复发组患者神经功能评分远低于无复发组。

（3）无复发组患者健康相关生命质量的各项评分的均值和标准差为：生理功能 38.93 ± 28.16 分，生理职能 30.05 ± 27.33 分，躯体疼痛 43.30 ± 20.62 分，总体健康 39.46 ± 21.96 分，活力 43.31 ± 20.62 分，社会功能 38.04 ± 27.72 分，情感职能 47.91 ± 24.50 分，精神健康 57.14 ± 19.12 分，生理健康总分 30.37 ± 25.58 分，心理健康总分 49.13 ± 18.98 分。与中国普通人群常模相比，无复发组患者各项分值明显下降，且生理健康总分下降程度比心理健康总分下降程度更明显。复发组患者得分远低于无复发组。

（4）患者的神经功能评分总分与生理健康总分呈高度正相关（$r=0.867$，$P < 0.001$），与心理健康总分呈中度正相关（$r=0.520$，$P=0.005$）。年龄、性别、社会经济地位评分、病理类型、出血量、手术并发症、手术入路等因素对健康相关生命质量的影响没有统计学差异。

（5）通过半结构化访谈发现：患者术后不能生活自理者 22 例，能生活自理者 11 例；患者术后社会交际明显减少者 28 例，社会交际基本正常者 5 例；患者术后无法继续上学或工作者 28 例，正常工作者 5 例；患者认为肿瘤及手术严重影响了家庭者 29 例，认为影响不大者 4 例；患者认为无法接受造瘘手术者 30 例，认为可以接受造瘘手术者 3 例；患者对术后康复指导有不同程度的需求者 33 例；患者对住院期间的医疗服务表示满意者 32 例，对住院期间的医疗服务表示不满者 1 例；患者对治疗结局表示满意者 23 例，对治疗结局表示不满者 10 例。

结论

全骶骨切除术治疗高位骶骨恶性肿瘤可以获得满意的肿瘤学切除边界，肿瘤学预后令人接受，但是手术并发症的发生率较高，并对患者造成了严重的神经功能损伤。

全骶骨切除术严重损害了患者的健康相关生命质量，总体上对患者生理健康的影响程度大于对心理健康的影响程度。患者的神经功能结局与健康相关生命质量呈明显的正相关。

全骶骨切除术对患者的生理、心理、社会和情感体验及其家庭造成了非常严重的影响。患者的术后康复需要更多的指导。同时患者基本上不愿意接受造瘘手术，认为没有必要同期行造瘘手术。

全骶骨切除术需严格把握适应证，并向患者充分告知手术的获益和潜在的风险，以便更好地做出手术决策，管理患者围手术期的预期，帮助患者康复。

关键词：全骶骨切除术；外科治疗结局；神经功能损伤；健康相关生命质量；定性分析

第 1 部分　骶骨常见恶性肿瘤的诊治

1　脊索瘤

1.1　定义

脊索是原脊椎动物的内部骨架。人类胚胎在发育的过程中，脊索逐渐形成一个中轴结构，一般在胚胎发育至 10 ～ 11 mm 时脊索完全发育成熟。之后脊索逐渐退化，伴随中轴骨多个骨化中心，脊索形成多个节段。胚胎发育至 2 个月时脊索变为椎间残留物，后面形成椎间盘的髓核。有时这种残留物可以出现在蝶枕区或骶尾部，或者椎体周围部分。在椎体中心，它们起源于未退化的椎间脊索管，可以形成较大的实体团块。脊索瘤好发于骶尾部和蝶枕区，是一种呈脊索样分化的肿瘤。

1.2　流行病学

脊索瘤占原发性恶性骨肿瘤的 3% ～ 4%，发病率较高，在骨肉瘤、软骨肉瘤和尤因肉瘤（Ewing 肉瘤）之后。脊索瘤好发于骶尾部和蝶枕区，多在 50 岁以上人群发病。美国国家癌症研究所癌症的监测、流行病学及结局（SEER）报告了1973—1987 年脊索瘤的发病率占所有原发性恶性骨肿瘤的 8.4%，且发病率随着年龄的增长而增加，50 ～ 60 岁为发病的高峰年龄段。20 岁以下发生脊索瘤的概率很低，该年龄段典型的发病部位是第 2 颈椎。脊索瘤首先好发于骶尾部和颅底，其次为颈椎和腰椎，再次为胸椎。脊索瘤大多起源于中轴骨。骶尾部脊索瘤可缓慢增长为巨大肿瘤，使骨外形膨胀，使医生难以辨认正常的解剖标志。脊索瘤一般呈溶骨性破坏，在脊柱可累及相邻 2 个或 2 个以上的椎体。骶尾部脊索瘤长大后可以压迫硬膜囊，尾骨的脊索瘤可以长向骶骨的前方和后方。

1.3　临床表现

疼痛是脊索瘤患者的主要症状，慢性疼痛持续加重，可持续几个月到几年。肿瘤增大后可压迫骶尾部神经，造成大小便功能障碍。脊索瘤往往表现为无痛性局部缓慢增长的肿瘤，晚期时可转移至肺部。

1.4 影像学表现

脊索瘤的 X 线片表现为溶骨性破坏，若脊索瘤内有钙化，在 X 线片上则表现为其内有散在的不透亮区域。CT（电子计算机断层扫描）检查能清楚显示肿瘤与周围组织（直肠、膀胱以及骶神经）的关系。核磁共振上脊索瘤表现为不均匀的高信号，并且可以清楚显示肿瘤破坏骨质以及压迫神经的情况。同位素扫描可以看到血液相和骨相同位素摄取均增高。血管造影可以清楚地显示肿瘤的血液供应。

1.5 病理表现

肉眼观察，可以看到脊索瘤有完整包膜的包块，其质软，一般不侵犯内脏。脊索瘤是灰褐色的分叶状实体瘤，呈胶状或黏液状。受累骨的表面有一层薄骨膜覆盖，术中操作容易使果冻样肿瘤流出，造成术野肿瘤扩散。复发的脊索瘤经常呈分叶状。脊索瘤增大后容易突入椎管，压迫脊髓和神经。

在显微镜下，能见到脊索瘤细胞胞浆空泡状的。可看到脊索瘤细胞内一个或几个空泡把细胞核挤到细胞的边上，因此又叫"印戒样"肿瘤细胞。典型的脊索瘤细胞较大，有位于中央的细胞核，有一层薄的胞浆在细胞核周围，在周边有胞浆空泡。因为胞浆大量空泡化，所以细胞呈透明形态。有些脊索瘤组织学呈肉瘤样表现，这是细胞核增长、不典型分裂所引起的。还有的看上去类似上皮来源肿瘤，这是空泡化不明显，嗜酸性染色胞浆深染造成的。

在电镜下，脊索瘤细胞胞浆的大部分区域由空泡样结构构成，并可见大量的高尔基体、粗面型内质网和糖原片状区域。脊索瘤细胞内可观察到由桥粒连接的中间丝。细胞外基质可观察到细小的低电子密度的颗粒状物质。脊索瘤细胞胞浆内可观察到微小管明显汇集。在免疫组化方面，S-100 蛋白和上皮性标志物（如细胞角蛋白和上皮膜抗原）在脊索瘤细胞表达为阳性。另外，神经丝染色和癌胚抗原（CEA）均有表达。与 Schiff 酸反应阳性的物质还可以在脊索瘤细胞胞浆中找到，这是检测淀粉糖化酶素的敏感物质。根据 DNA 多倍体检测结果发现，脊索瘤染色体可能是非整倍体或二倍体。以上这些研究结论的临床意义及其与肿瘤生物学行为的关系还需进一步研究。

1.6 鉴别诊断

脊索瘤需与软骨肉瘤鉴别。在脊索瘤中，细胞典型表现是空泡样细胞索条状排列以及黏液样基质。普通软骨肉瘤中也可出现类似细胞的条索状排列和黏液样基质，不同的是，软骨肉瘤 S-100 蛋白染色呈阳性而上皮性标志物染色呈阴性。

其他黏液样骨肿瘤，如软骨黏液性纤维瘤，一般不易与脊索瘤混淆，因为它极少累及中轴骨。有时脊索瘤容易与上皮来源的肿瘤混淆，特别是细胞丰富并结合成细胞袖，同时细胞核不呈典型分裂的组织。此外，脊索瘤需与转移性腺癌鉴别，因其广泛的透明细胞样或印戒细胞样形态，还需联系临床与影像学表现来帮助鉴别。必须指出的是，有时在其他肿瘤比如转移性腺癌检测时，也可以出现共同表达 S-100 蛋白和上皮性标志物。

1.7 治疗方法

脊索瘤经常呈局部进展性生长，局部复发率较高。骶尾部脊索瘤通常会影响重要的器官并导致死亡。为了达到良好的局部控制和预防肿瘤转移，建议行广泛的大块切除手术。如果为了保留神经功能而仅仅行边缘切除，脊索瘤非常容易复发。囊内刮除则基本没有作用，不建议进行。脊索瘤平均生存期约 4 年，死亡率较高，很少有患者生存超过 10 年。近年来，随着医疗技术的进步，脊索瘤患者总体生存率有了明显提高。SEER 对 1973—1987 年脊索瘤的统计数据表明，脊索瘤患者的 5 年生存率由 1973 年的 40% 提高到了 1987 年的 65%。治疗上应尽可能完全切除脊索瘤，不能完全切除的脊索瘤可行减瘤术和辅助放疗。不同研究报道的脊索瘤转移率差别较大，平均转移率为 40%。有些高转移率报道包括了脊索瘤复发造成的局部转移。真正远处转移率小于 10%。累及多骨或同时累及软组织是脊索瘤复发的高危因素。脊索瘤远处转移一般是肺，也会有局部淋巴结的转移，多见于病程晚期。在少数情况下，脊索瘤临床早期出现远处转移和大量瘤栓栓塞血管，这表明部分脊索瘤出现侵袭性较强的生物学行为。放疗不能防止脊索瘤细胞转移，但可以暂时控制肿瘤的局部生长。不过不建议行术前放疗，也不建议行化疗，因为脊索瘤对化疗不敏感。

2 恶性骨巨细胞肿瘤

2.1 定义

骨巨细胞瘤中的恶性肿瘤，叫恶性骨巨细胞瘤或去分化的巨细胞瘤，是一种来源于巨细胞的高度恶性的肿瘤，是原发或者发生在之前发生过巨细胞肿瘤部位的肉瘤。

2.2 流行病学

骨巨细胞肿瘤的恶性肿瘤大多发生在骨巨细胞瘤放疗治疗之后，原发的恶性骨巨细胞肿瘤非常少。实际上发生恶性转变的骨巨细胞肿瘤发病率只有不到 1%，女性发病率略高于男性。恶性骨巨细胞瘤的发病年龄比骨巨细胞瘤的大 10 岁左右。如果骨巨细胞瘤在治疗后出现恶变，往往表现为反复发生的疼痛和肿胀。

2.3　临床表现

恶性骨巨细胞肿瘤的病程长短不一，大多数在半年以上，数周至数年不等。主要症状表现为疼痛、肿胀、包块，少数病例表现为外伤后的疼痛。肿块增大有 3 种情况：①发生病理性骨折后形成巨大肿块；②逐渐增大；③在短时间内迅速增大。肿块局部会伴有静脉怒张、皮温升高、压痛，关节附近的肿块往往会导致关节活动受限。

2.4　影像学表现

在 X 线上，恶性骨巨细胞肿瘤表现为广泛溶骨性破坏，骨骺、干骺端的破坏，这种破坏可以蔓延至附近的骨干，残端类似溶冰，可以完全溶骨。成分房状膨胀的骨质破坏，骨皮质呈薄壳状菲薄膨胀，破坏区常表现为分房状或泡沫状溶骨性破坏，溶骨性破坏可侵入关节，破坏关节软骨。恶性骨巨细胞肿瘤可以导致骨皮质破坏，穿入软组织形成巨大肿块。在 X 线片上，软组织阴影内肿块一般呈无骨化或钙化征象。恶性骨巨细胞肿瘤可出现骨膜反应，呈现类似 Codman 三角或葱皮样骨膜反应的表现。

2.5　病理表现

在大体标本，继发恶性骨巨细胞瘤和高度恶性的肉瘤非常相似，可以观察到大块的鱼肉样白色肿瘤组织，且往往伴有软组织肿块。如果是原发恶性骨巨细胞瘤，一般可在骨端发现暗红色或黄褐色的肿块。在组织病理学上，继发的恶性骨巨细胞瘤，类似于高度恶性的梭形细胞肉瘤，表现为肿瘤细胞产生或者不产生骨样组织。而在原发恶性骨巨细胞瘤中，可以观察到传统意义上的巨细胞瘤的圆形或卵圆形的单核细胞和多核的巨细胞，还可以看到核异型性的梭形细胞，但是有时观察不到多核的巨细胞。

2.6　鉴别诊断与分型

恶性骨巨细胞肿瘤的诊断强调临床检查、X 线检查和病理检查三结合。恶性骨巨细胞瘤的诊断必须十分谨慎，此诊断需在同一瘤内有典型骨巨细胞瘤和肉瘤组织相并存，或以前曾在同一部位确定是良性骨巨细胞瘤。观察表明，在其他骨肿瘤与瘤样病变的组织中，有时也可以观察到类似于骨巨细胞瘤中基质细胞、多核巨细胞的形态，因此需注意鉴别诊断。鉴别诊断主要与溶骨性骨肉瘤、骨纤维肉瘤和骨恶性纤维组织细胞瘤等其他溶骨性肉瘤鉴别。

根据临床特点，将恶性骨巨细胞瘤分为两型：①原发型：指骨巨细胞瘤开始治疗后1年内诊断为恶性者；②转变型：此型又分为a、b两个亚型，a型肿瘤指在开始治疗后超过1年但在5年内被诊断为恶性者；b型肿瘤指在开始治疗后超过5年被诊断为恶性者。某学者将恶性骨巨细胞瘤分为三型：①原发型：指一开始为恶性者；②演变型：指良性骨巨细胞瘤在短期内演变为恶性者；③继发型：指良性骨巨细胞瘤在相对的无症状期后，通常在放疗后继发为恶性者。也有学者按组织学分型将恶性骨巨细胞瘤分为两型：①纤维肉瘤的毛细血管扩张型，原发者多为此型；②纤维肉瘤的呈胶原型，继发者多见。

2.7 治疗方法

施行广泛性手术是主要的治疗方案，可以辅助化疗，如行截肢术、关节离断术等根治术，这样可以达到治愈的目的，而对于不能切除的肿瘤，则建议采用放疗作为姑息治疗。恶性骨巨细胞瘤的预后并不好，但稍好于骨肉瘤、尤因肉瘤（Ewing肉瘤）。恶性骨巨细胞瘤生存率比其他溶骨性表现的肉瘤生存率高，因此治疗的首要目的是彻底切除肿瘤、防止肿瘤复发及转移，同时尽量保留肢体功能。根治术适用于病程短、早期侵犯软组织，并向四周扩散，瘤体巨大，肢体无法保留者。如果肿瘤发生于骨内，未穿破骨皮质及软组织，术中冰冻切片病理结果为恶性，则建议行肿瘤段切除术，术后建议辅助放疗。化疗对恶性骨巨细胞瘤的疗效还不明确，需要进一步观察以积累经验。继发性的恶性骨巨细胞瘤预后比原发性的恶性骨巨细胞瘤预后要好，其类似于高度恶性的梭形细胞肉瘤预后。

3 骨肉瘤

3.1 定义

骨肉瘤是一种高度恶性肿瘤，原发于骨髓内，其典型特征为增殖的肿瘤细胞直接形成骨或骨样组织，因此又叫作骨肉瘤。骨肉瘤常起源于骨内，由产生骨质的间质细胞产生，也是最常发生在骨的原发性恶性肿瘤。

3.2　流行病学

就所有肿瘤整体而言，骨肉瘤并不太常见，但就骨的原发性恶性骨肿瘤而言，骨肉瘤是最常见的。在人类的恶性肿瘤中，每年每一百万人中有 2～3 例。典型骨肉瘤男性发病率高于女性，男女比约为（1.5～2）∶1。绝大多数病例在 10～30 岁发病，少数见于 10 岁前及 30 岁之后。骨肉瘤的好发部位依次为股骨远端、胫骨近端、肱骨近端（这 3 个部位发病率的比例约为 4∶2∶1）。骨肉瘤常发病于长骨的干骺端，极少数病例发生于脊柱或骶骨。

骨肉瘤病程短、进展快，有时肿瘤可在数日内明显增大膨出，出现局部跳跃灶。骨肉瘤迅猛生长大多由肿瘤出血所致。也有少部分骨肉瘤缓慢生长，其症状隐匿，潜伏 1 年以上，一般表现为硬化成骨。骨肉瘤最常见的转移部位是肺，晚期可转移至骨，在发生骨转移时，一般已经发生肺部转移。骨肉瘤一般向肺或骨转移，很少转移到内脏。局部区域性淋巴结转移在骨肉瘤中非常罕见。

3.3　临床表现

大多数骨肉瘤患者在起病初期无典型临床表现。在起病初期，患者仅有围绕膝关节的疼痛，呈中等程度并间歇发作，且活动后疼痛加剧。此时很容易被漏诊或者误诊，由于患者多处于青春期或青壮年期，身体健壮，且经常参加体育活动，一旦出现疼痛极易被误诊为创伤，或被误诊为风湿性病变，便会行抗风湿治疗。在骨肉瘤初期，临床医师很少考虑进行放射性检查的必要。

发病后在数周内，患者疼痛可逐渐加重，然后持续发作。局部可在早期出现疼痛、肿胀的表现。肿瘤肿胀一般非常迅速，少部分相对缓慢。由于肿瘤本身血供丰富，肿块局部皮温常增高，伴局部明显触痛。在骨肉瘤病变进展变快时，一般会出现肿瘤附近的关节功能障碍，局部软组织浸润发红，出现局部水肿及明显的浅表静脉网状怒张。少数病例出现骨质溶解，当其进展迅猛时，可在疼痛部位并发病理骨折，但并不多见。少数情况下，当骨肉瘤累及骨面时，关节腔内可有积液渗出，出现关节积液。局部淋巴结很少出现转移，但在肿瘤进展显著时，这种病例常可发生淋巴结炎。

在初次确诊时，患者很少出现恶液质，一般情况比较良好。患者开始出现肺转移或骨转移时，就会出现体重下降和贫血现象。从首发症状到治疗的时间，一般不多于 6 个月，少数患者发病 1 年以上才接受治疗。

3.4 影像学表现

在 X 线上，骨肉瘤破坏性和渗透性很强，表现为侵袭性，能产生骨或骨样组织，X 线透亮区为侵袭和破坏区的特征，肿瘤很快会破坏皮质骨并进入软组织，因此分界不清楚，但较少会跨越骨骺板和骨骺，不会进入关节腔。反应骨的 Codman 三角一般在皮质骨穿透区，而病变边缘一般无反应骨。有时可观察到病变的其他部位有不定型的非应力定向的瘤性骨，这是骨肉瘤不完全矿化导致的。如果新生骨与长骨纵轴呈直角，可以表现为日光放射线状，这种现象曾被认定是骨肉瘤的独特表现，但近期发现在其他一些恶性肿瘤也有类似表现，因此，日光放射线并非骨肉瘤的特有表现。

骨肉瘤在 X 线上可有 3 种表现：①成骨性，主要表现为不透过放射线的影像；②溶骨性，以 X 线透亮为主；③混合性，两种 X 线表现均存在。三者在临床进程或预后无差异。即使术前化疗效果比较满意，也很少观察到肿块显著减小，不过患者疼痛明显减轻，而且 X 线上可以观察到肿块减小或停止生长，同时可以观察到病灶内原透亮区骨化增加，软组织肿块周围反应骨壳形成。

骨肉瘤病变区域的骨代谢很强，因此放射性核素骨扫描可显示活跃形成的矿化骨有很强的摄取能力，并能很清楚地显示骨肉瘤化疗前后病变的发展和变化。同时，可检查骨肉瘤有无其他骨转移灶及跳跃病灶存在。

CT 扫描可补充放射性核素扫描和血管造影的材料，为骨肉瘤的诊断提供更准确的信息。CT 扫描用于明确骨肉瘤髓内和软组织肿块范围，且比 X 线更敏感。在髓腔内 CT 值的增高一般提示已有骨肉瘤的浸润，并能及早发现骨肉瘤髓腔内跳跃灶。CT 对病变瘤骨的显示优于 X 线和磁共振成像（MRI），这是由于骨肉瘤病变骨周边部分的骨化弱于中央部分的，CT 扫描可敏感地分辨较弱成骨的周边部分，MRI 通常不易区分信号相近的骨肉瘤弱成骨区和未成骨区。肺部 CT 扫描是确认骨肉瘤有无肺转移灶的最好方法。

磁共振检查能够很好地显示骨肉瘤的髓内范围、跳跃灶，同时可以观察软组织肿块范围及是否侵及骨骺或关节，骨肉瘤在 T1 加权像为低信号，在 T2 加权像的信号较 T1 时强，但比脂肪、液体信号弱。

血管造影能描绘出骨肉瘤病变软组织部分边缘的反应性新生血管区，反应区可显示早期动脉扩张。血管造影虽不能显示骨肉瘤特异性组织的发生，但可以表明骨肉瘤的高血运状态。通过骨扫描，可以明确肿瘤侵犯的范围，某些骨肉瘤病例不能通过骨扫描发现转移至其他部位的肿瘤和跳跃灶。

3.5　活检

骨肉瘤的活检应该在初步的评估结束后马上进行。无论是闭合的穿刺活检还是开放地切开活检，都可以获得病理诊断标本。如果临床表现和影像学表现都提示为比较典型的骨肉瘤，建议使用穿刺活检；当有明显的软组织肿块时，穿刺活检一般也比较容易获取病理标本。

穿刺活检有其局限性和缺点。最终手术时需要切除针道穿刺点，因此穿刺点必须位于最终手术的切口线部位。切开活检是最常用的活检方法，它的优点是可以获得较多的组织，病理医师不仅可以用这些组织做常规的病理检查，还有足够的标本进行流式细胞 DNA 测量和细胞遗传学等其他检查。

3.6　病理表现

在大体标本上，骨肉瘤的外观表现多种多样，这和肿瘤发生的部位、肿瘤骨质及反应骨质形成的多少、原有骨质破坏及出血的程度、坏死灶的范围等因素都有关系。部分骨肉瘤还可以观察到软骨形成区。骨肉瘤大体切开后切面上瘤组织底色一般为灰红色，黄白色明显处是骨肉瘤肿瘤骨质形成的部位，半透明区是骨肉瘤形成软骨的部位，坏死灶显示为灰黄色，出血区显示为暗红色。一般同一骨肉瘤瘤体内这几种不同颜色混合，构成骨肉瘤大体标本多彩状的特点，若以某一种颜色为主要表现，则说明以某一成分为主。以前认为，成骨性骨肉瘤是以成骨为主的骨肉瘤，溶骨性骨肉瘤是以溶骨为主、原有骨组织被大量破坏且出血坏死较多的骨肉瘤，但实际上上述两种表现常见于同一瘤体的不同部分。骨肉瘤的肿瘤骨质一般可如象牙样，明显广泛现于中央部，而在瘤体外部较少见。骨肉瘤瘤骨丰富的部位质地硬实，瘤骨稀少部位则质软具沙砾感或如鱼肉样。长骨骨肉瘤一般在干骺端，可侵及骨髓腔及向一侧或四周骨质浸润，有时可于一处或多处穿透骨皮质将骨膜掀起，有时向周围软组织生长形成结节状或梭形包块。骨肉瘤所产生的骨质，可以形成数条放射状排列的骨质条索，由骨皮质表层向外伸展，与骨干纵轴垂直或斜行，形成日光放射线征象。常有大量的骨组织增殖在被骨组织掀起的骨膜下，表现为 Codman 三角。当骨肉瘤进一步扩展时，Codman 三角因边界不清而消失。

骨肉瘤生长迅速，一方面可以向髓腔及骨皮质扩展并侵及骨膜和软组织；另一方面，骨肉瘤可向骨骺蔓延，破坏骨骺后，骨肉瘤肿瘤组织可以侵及关节软骨。少数骨肉瘤组织可越过关节软骨侵入关节囊。骨肉瘤可在原发肿瘤同一骨内另一处形成孤立性转移结节，转移至邻近关节对侧的骨内，形成孤立性的转移结节，即在骨内可呈跳跃灶。此种转移一般是肿瘤组织通过关节旁丰富的小静脉吻合支或骨髓内血窦转移的。

骨肉瘤能直接产生肿瘤性骨样组织和骨组织，在镜下可以观察到骨肉瘤由明显间变的瘤细胞组成。骨肉瘤细胞大小不一，有丰富的染色质，呈粗颗粒或凝块状，有明显增大的核仁和病理性分裂象。如果骨肉瘤组织分化差，则可以观察到肿瘤性骨质稀少区，瘤细胞异型性较显著。在肿瘤骨形成量较多的区域，可以观察到瘤细胞异型性相对较轻。肿瘤性骨质一般不形成板层骨，表现为骨样组织或网状骨质。骨肉瘤瘤骨最早形成是在恶性瘤细胞间出现胶原样物质，呈同质性淡红色，此时需与胶原纤维的透明变性鉴别。骨肉瘤组织在 VanGieson（VG）染色呈红染，但观察其波纹状及编织状结构，发现骨肉瘤组织周围并无明显纤维化，可见到恶性瘤细胞。有时可以在一些骨肉瘤组织观察到钙盐颗粒沉着，其内瘤细胞固缩变小，形成肿瘤性骨质钙化。骨肉瘤的肿瘤性骨样组织和骨质分布也不均匀，量多少不一，多者可以观察到大片瘤细胞散在其中，少者可以观察到大片瘤细胞间的小碎粒状。骨肉瘤的典型组织学特点是肿瘤性骨样组织构成纤维不规则编织状或绸带交织状。

当骨肉瘤肿瘤性骨质越多并有形成骨小梁结构倾向时，其病灶内的瘤细胞数目也明显减少、分散，瘤细胞趋向较成熟的骨细胞，可观察到瘤细胞有异型性，这是分化高的肿瘤性骨质，并非反应性骨质。若骨肉瘤组织正常骨质已被破坏溶解，则很少观察到残留正常骨小梁，瘤骨形成较少。若正常骨质未被破坏溶解，则瘤骨形成明显，原有骨小梁结构仍可保留。这些残留正常的骨小梁骨细胞，虽然数量少，但是分布均匀，尽管多已坏死仅留下空虚的陷窝，但骨小梁也可被周围的瘤细胞所蚕食致使形态不规则，或被瘤骨包绕或与之连接，形成瘤骨间的支架。骨肉瘤病变组织常可见有多核瘤巨细胞，有深染的细胞核，有明显的异型性，细胞核的大小形态奇特，细胞核多为 3～5 个，核仁明显增大。有时可观察到破骨细胞型多核巨细胞，这是机体对骨肉瘤组织免疫反应的表现，机体发挥参与溶解正常或肿瘤性骨质的作用，而不是肿瘤细胞成分。有些部位破骨细胞型多核巨细胞较多，难以和骨巨细胞瘤鉴别。此时需注意这类巨细胞的细胞核不具异型性，由此与肿瘤性多核巨细胞作鉴别。

骨肉瘤组织有一个特点，即组织化学或细胞化学碱性磷酸酶（AKP）均呈强阳性反应。不管是瘤细胞还是瘤巨细胞，在胞浆外缘 AKP 活性较明显，AKP 在肿瘤外围生长活跃区活性最高。骨化不明显处 AKP 表达呈阳性，AKP 活性低或呈阴性往往是埋在类骨质或编织骨内的瘤细胞，因此 AKP 在骨质硬化区的表达比瘤细胞丰富区明显减弱。

3.7 鉴别诊断

3.7.1 骨髓炎

骨髓炎好发于儿童和青少年，是一种常见病。儿童好发于骨骺端，成年人也可出现，多见于胫骨上端、股骨下端、肱骨和桡骨。骨髓炎病变一般不易越过骨骺线，最常见的细菌感染为金黄色葡萄球菌感染，主要的临床症状包括局部软组织肿胀、疼痛、不愿活动患肢，局部深压痛，常伴有全身发热。血常规提示白细胞总数和中性粒细胞数明显增加，红细胞沉降率（血沉）测定和 C 反应蛋白明显增高。一般可行分层穿刺，若能抽出脓液或血性液，在显微镜下观察到脓球即可确诊。X 线表现一般晚于临床症状，早期可出现骨膜反应，并伴随局部软组织肿胀，晚期可出现网格状骨密度降低，溶骨性破坏。破坏骨边缘清楚，新生骨密度升高，骨膜反应光滑完整。骨破坏区看不到成骨反应，成骨区看不到骨溶解。如骨破坏广泛，则有死骨形成，常有向骨干发展倾向。

3.7.2 尤因肉瘤

尤因肉瘤发病年龄一般低于 20 岁，发病部位是股骨远端、胫骨近端，一般表现为间歇性疼痛转为持续性，进行性加重。软组织肿块可在早期出现，密度较高，肿块随病变进展越来越明显。在 X 线可以观察到层状或葱皮状骨膜增生，骨干骨髓腔呈斑片状溶骨性破坏，可以观察到明显的骨破坏。尤因肉瘤的特征性改变始于一侧皮质病变时，因皮质内面完整而皮质表面被侵蚀而形成蝶形，肿瘤髓内生长破坏皮质由内向外变薄，直至消失。尤因肉瘤的骨膜增生常呈纺锤状，中心性骨质被破坏、无死骨，肿瘤周围新骨增生，可以观察到 Codman 三角表现。尤因肉瘤因高度恶性致使转移较早，故放射线治疗有效。

3.7.3 骨纤维肉瘤

骨纤维肉瘤好发于骨干，表现为溶骨性肿瘤，其发病年龄比骨肉瘤的大，属于成纤维性结缔组织肉瘤。病理组织可观察到纵横交错的胶原纤维束，而缺乏其他组织分化。在 X 线片可以观察到溶骨性破坏，呈束状或斑片状，在髓腔呈偏心性生长；可以观察到少量骨膜下新骨或骨膜三角，软组织肿块一般不大，很少有新骨形成。此病常常发生病理性骨折。

3.8 治疗方法

目前，骨肉瘤一般需要行综合治疗，即手术和化疗联合治疗。在 20 世纪 80 年代前，治疗手段以截肢为主，治疗效果极差，患者的 5 年生存率仅为 10% ～ 20%。90 年代以后逐渐开展手术后辅助化疗，21 世纪以后逐渐开展新辅助化疗，即术前化疗—手术—术后化疗，治疗效果较前明显改善。

3.8.1 截肢术

截肢术是目前临床上治疗骨肉瘤的重要手段之一，包括高位截肢术和关节离断术。截肢手术操作相对简单，无需特别的技术和设备，能最大限度地切除原发病灶，术后可尽快施行化疗控制肿瘤转移。但截肢术导致患者永久丧失肢体，严重影响患者的生活质量。另外，截肢术后常常合并幻肢痛，有些患者受到慢性、长期的幻肢痛影响，患者的心理健康和生理健康受到严重影响，生活质量严重下降。

3.8.2 保肢术

保肢术能够保留肢体，但有严格的适应证：①属于 Enneking 分期 A 期或对化疗反应好的 B 期，主要表现是神经、血管未受累；②全身情况及局部软组织条件允许，可以达到广泛性切除；③无转移病灶或转移病灶可以治愈；④患者有强烈的保肢愿望；⑤经济上能承受高强度的化疗。手术方案的选择，主要看肿瘤的分期与肿瘤对化疗的反应，尤其是后者更为重要，新辅助化疗的有效实施及良好的化疗反应是保肢术的关键环节。保肢术的手术方式种类较多，主要包括假体置换、灭活再植、关节融合、生物性关节成形、异体骨移植等。

3.8.3 化疗

20世纪70年代，有学者开始对骨肉瘤进行手术后化疗，称为辅助化疗，常用的化疗药物包括阿霉素（doxorubicin，DOX）、顺铂（cisplatin，CDP）、氨甲蝶呤（methotrexate，MTX）。1982年，Rosen 等又提出在手术前进行化疗即新辅助化疗，可以缩小肿瘤体积，为保肢术提供条件。术后评估化疗敏感性，对标本进行肿瘤坏死率检查。

总之，骨肉瘤需要进行综合治疗，以外科手术为主，化疗为辅，肿瘤细胞对化疗的敏感度直接影响其生存率，所以系统、正规的化疗非常关键。术前化疗—手术—术后化疗的模式已在全国进行推广，骨肉瘤患者的生存率较以前有较大提高。目前，骨肉瘤的治疗已进入平台期，新的骨肉瘤治疗方法尚未出现。随着肿瘤生长、侵袭性的分子水平实验研究和临床研究越来越深入，骨肉瘤治疗的平台期将会得到进一步突破。新药的开发、剂量强化、多药耐药性的克服、放射增敏剂及生物调节、免疫、基因治疗等为骨肉瘤的治疗提供了新的靶点。

3.9 预后情况

20世纪80年代的一些研究表明，对于局限的可切除的肢体骨肉瘤单行手术治疗与1970年以前的治疗结果相同，即确诊后6个月内50%以上的患者出现肿瘤转移，确诊后 2 年 80% 以上的患者再次出现肿瘤，单纯手术后能够无瘤生存的患者低于 20%。而近 20 年来，骨肉瘤的治疗效果取得了巨大的进步。利用先进的影像学检查（如 CT、MRI）能够清晰地显示肿瘤的局部解剖情况和生长方式。胸部螺旋 CT 扫描可发现隐匿的肺转移。另外，改良的分级系统有助于判断患者的预后情况。多药联合化疗极大地提高了患者的施行保肢术的可能性和长期生存率。其他方面也取得了明显进步，比如假体的设计和对异体骨使用经验的积累等，使肢体骨肉瘤患者的保肢手术率提高至 90% ～ 95%。目前，经过正规的化疗—手术—化疗，患者 5 年生存率可达到 60% ～ 80%。

4　软骨肉瘤

4.1　定义

软骨肉瘤是常见的原发恶性骨肿瘤，是一种恶性结缔组织肿瘤，其细胞有向软骨分化、形成软骨基质的特点。

4.2　流行病学

软骨肉瘤约占原发恶性骨肿瘤的 10%，男性发病率高于女性（约 2：1），好发于 30 ～ 70 岁。软骨肉瘤好发于扁骨、长管状骨的近端，而发生于脊柱或骶骨的并不多。

4.3　临床表现

软骨肉瘤早期症状为隐袭性的疼痛，等肿瘤已生长到较大后才发现肿块。如果肿瘤发生于盆腔等有较大空间的部位，只有肿瘤体积达到一定水平时临床上才能发现。因此，软骨肉瘤一般表现症状轻微、发展缓慢，且病程较长，通常呈间歇性发作的深部轻微疼痛。早期肿瘤未侵犯软组织，一般不能触及肿块，晚期常可形成大的、能触及的软组织肿块。发生在脊柱、骶骨的软骨肉瘤可因压迫脊髓、神经而出现相应的神经根性疼痛或功能障碍。若肿瘤生长迅速且呈侵袭性，早期即可破坏骨皮质并侵犯软组织，应考虑为去分化征象或是肿瘤恶性升级。偶尔有肿瘤经骺端侵入关节，引起关节症状，病理性骨折较少见。有时术后复发的软骨肉瘤可表现出比原发肿瘤更强的侵袭性。

4.4　影像学表现

软骨肉瘤在 X 线片上的典型表现为骨内溶骨性破坏，并伴有大量钙化，在骨干为中心性生长，在干骺端为偏心生长。软骨肉瘤一般生长缓慢，偶尔很快。如果长骨发生软骨肉瘤且生长缓慢，可观察到特征性的髓腔膨胀，外侧骨皮质可变薄，内侧骨膜受到肿瘤侵犯，表现为扇贝样花边状改变。骨皮质在较长的时间缓慢发生反应性骨化增生反应，表现为骨皮质增厚，一般无骨膜反应。若肿瘤呈明显侵袭性发展，则能观察到边缘模糊的骨溶解区，可伴有或不伴有骨皮质的破坏。X线检查可表现为肿瘤内不透光性增加，这是因为软骨有钙化及骨化的倾向。软骨钙化的特征性改变，在X线上可表现为结节状、环形钙化，或无结构的、不规则散布的喷雾状颗粒。若骨壳内有骨脊形成，可表现为泡沫状或面包屑样改变。病灶钙化较致密时，可使肿瘤呈现出不透光改变。在极少数情况下，肿瘤可侵袭松质骨，使得局部钙盐沉积，出现反应性骨化，松质骨密度均匀增高，肿瘤的骨内部分在X线上仍不显影，需要结合骨扫描CT、MRI检查结果加以诊断。软骨肉瘤恶性程度越高，钙化越少，在低度恶性的高分化软骨肉瘤中则钙化较多。

因为阻力相对较小，软骨肉瘤往往向骨干的髓腔浸润生长。在约近半数的X线图像上显示肿瘤已浸润扩展至整个长骨的1/3、1/2或更广泛的部位。但肿瘤开始侵入髓腔时在X线上可能不明显。通常应用骨扫描、CT及MRI等检查全面研究和确定肿瘤在髓腔内的范围。CT和MRI检查可以进一步了解肿瘤在骨及软组织中的范围，是明确早期中心型软骨肉瘤的主要检查手段之一。在CT上，软骨肉瘤一般呈现为伴有散在高密度钙化的髓内肿块，呈分叶状。在MRI上，软骨肉瘤呈非特异性表现，一般在T1加权像上为低到中信号，在T2加权像上为高信号，整个肿瘤为分页状，钙化灶为低信号表现。增强MRI可看到扇贝样花边状的强化。

软骨肉瘤在放射线同位素扫描上主要表现为浓集现象，而且同位素聚集的范围常常大于肿瘤的实际边界，这是邻近组织充血水肿引起的敏感性增高。骨扫描还可发现潜在的转移肿瘤病灶。

4.5 病理表现

软骨肉瘤是由肿瘤细胞产生的恶性软骨，有时不太容易评估软骨肿瘤的恶性程度。软骨肉瘤有多种分型和分级系统，其中病理分级广为接受，且对普通软骨肉瘤预后有指导意义。其分级标准主要是根据细胞的多少，细胞核的大小、分裂象及异型性，由此可将软骨肉瘤分为三级：Ⅰ级软骨肉瘤具有分化良好的透明软骨，异型细胞较少；Ⅱ级具有较多的细胞成分，比Ⅰ级软骨肉瘤有更多的间变特征；Ⅲ级软骨肉瘤恶性度较高，肿瘤细胞成分丰富，异型性明显。

　　肉眼观察下，Ⅰ级的低度恶性中心型软骨肉瘤，骨皮质可表现正常或轻度膨胀而无肿瘤浸润。低度恶性中心型软骨肉瘤的表现与软骨瘤的并无太大差别。如果肿瘤长期缓慢生长，可能破坏骨皮质而长成大的肿瘤。Ⅱ～Ⅲ级中央型软骨肉瘤的骨皮质经常被肿瘤侵袭破坏，在肿瘤的一些区域可观察到分化良好的软骨，常可形成相互紧密贴连的小叶。软骨肉瘤的软骨比正常的软骨和软骨瘤更为灰暗、柔软、湿润，且更加透明。在黏液区，可以观察到胶样状态和灰白色的组织，有时可观察到黏液样液化区和出血区。在骨内及血供不良的中央型软骨肉瘤新鲜组织中，还可以观察到因供血不足而出现变性坏死的组织。肿瘤切面可以观察到白色、不透明的坏死部分及囊性或出血性液化，有时还可以看到钙盐沉积，质地硬，有类似沙砾感，钙化常以颗粒状或点状分布，围绕软骨小叶周围。骨肉瘤等高度恶性肿瘤可直接侵蚀破坏骨皮质，但大多数中心型软骨肉瘤常向阻力较小的哈弗氏系统浸润生长，发生慢性成骨反应，一般仅导致骨皮质外侧增厚。软骨肉瘤在未穿透骨皮质前，可在髓腔内向骨干扩展很长的距离。在某些软骨肉瘤中，肿瘤可侵及关节。

　　在显微镜下，分级不同的软骨肉瘤表现不同。Ⅰ级软骨肉瘤发生率大约占20%，它有分化良好的软骨，有黏液区。区别于软骨瘤的细胞特征包括以下几点：①细胞核轻度增大；②细胞核大多为圆形，大小不等；③可见双核细胞；④细胞数多。Ⅱ级软骨肉瘤发生率占60%，最为常见。软骨组织表现明显的异型性，细胞核大，且染色深；双核细胞十分普遍，三核细胞则少见；有些细胞核大小可为正常细胞核的 4～5 倍，且形态奇异。软骨肉瘤组织可以部分或全部呈黏液样，肿瘤细胞呈梭形，有时呈圆形，它们散在或聚集成小群，或是多层状重叠。细胞胞浆透明，有丰富的黏液伴轻度的嗜碱性基质。可见细胞核异型性，可观察到肥大而深染的细胞核，有时呈双核，偶可见有丝分裂象。Ⅱ级中心型软骨肉瘤常常广泛浸润宿主骨的髓腔，被浸润的骨小梁可不被破坏，当肿瘤已侵入软组织时可有假包膜围绕而有明确界限。但假包膜本身也可被新生物的卫星灶所浸润。Ⅲ级软骨肉瘤发生率占20%，它几乎总是有分化好的软骨，然而软骨小叶的边缘都由致密的成软骨细胞及未分化的间质成分组成致使其颜色深染。软骨细胞很不典型，数量多，以明显异型性及细胞核深染为特点，它们通常为巨核，为正常细胞核的 5～10 倍，细胞有 3 个或多个细胞核且核形怪异，可见到有丝分裂象。Ⅲ级中心型软骨肉瘤迅速而广泛地浸润周围骨，并破坏骨质，在软组织内它也表现出明显的浸润性。

　　中心型软骨肉瘤的组织学分级与它的病程及预后明显相关，因此软骨肉瘤分级在确定治疗计划时有很高的参考价值。区别软骨瘤和Ⅰ级软骨肉瘤与确定软骨肉瘤之间的分级同样是比较困难的，需要考虑以下几个方面：①组织学的取材和观察必须以肿瘤的活跃区为重点，而不是软骨钙化、骨化的区域。从这些钙化、骨化区域无法评估病变区域的细胞学恶性程度。②整个肿瘤的细胞恶性特征不均一，不同区域有很大差别，因此，组织学标本越多越好。检查者应观察标本的所有区域，那些显示高度恶性特征的区域才能确定肿瘤的组织学特征，以及作为恶性度分级依据。③在细胞学恶性特征表现不明显时，一定要结合临床资料、影像学表现及肉眼所见加以分析。例如：轻度细胞核多形、细胞核肥大和深染、细胞双核，并不表明恶性。如果软骨瘤位于手的管状骨或为软骨瘤病的一部分，尤其发生在儿童时期（软骨肉瘤很少发生于青春期前）或是骨膜软骨瘤，这些病例的细胞学表现可能更加不典型，类似于Ⅱ级软骨肉瘤的表现，而结果不表明恶性。相反，如果软骨性肿瘤位于主要长骨或躯干骨，即使只有轻微的非典型性增生表现，也要考虑到局部复发及恶性的可能性。同样地，在出现临床及放射学表现明显生长，无病理骨折而有疼痛，和骨扫描阳性初次切除后复发致使的肿瘤体积增大，有贝壳样膨胀改变甚至超越骨皮质时应考虑诊断为中心型软骨肉瘤，而不是软骨瘤。

坏死、钙化和骨化现象在所有的软骨肉瘤中都很普遍。软骨肉瘤中的骨化由新生骨组成，无恶性特征。这是用修复骨来替代退化的及钙化的软骨，或仅是内骨膜或外骨膜对肿瘤侵犯的反应骨。从无间质细胞直接产生类骨质，若是这样就诊断为骨肉瘤。

4.6 诊断与鉴别诊断

4.6.1 诊断

诊断软骨肉瘤时，应综合研究和评估临床及影像学资料。具有同样组织学表现的软骨性肿瘤诊断为良性或恶性，取决于患者年龄、发生部位、症状表现、放射学检查、骨扫描和CT特征等情况。在组织学上，必须通过整个肿瘤至少一个横断面的切片检查后才能确定软骨肉瘤的恶性程度。软骨肉瘤通常生长缓慢，症状多但不严重，且常发生于松质骨处，躯干及肢带骨放射学上难以发现，早期诊断较困难，所以常被误诊为肩周炎、腰椎间盘突出症、骨性关节病等。也有发生在骨盆或股骨近端的软骨肉瘤，长期不能经检查发现者。因此，当30岁以上的患者，有持续性轻到中度疼痛症状又不能用普通的关节病或神经综合征解释，且对相应治疗无反应时，应进行骨扫描、CT和MRI检查，以排除软骨肉瘤的可能。因为手术是治疗软骨肉瘤的唯一手段，所以对肿瘤的分级必须准确。为进一步明确诊断，术前应仔细进行活检，以制订合适的手术治疗方案。

4.6.2　鉴别诊断

鉴别诊断中，最为困难的是低度恶性或临界性软骨肉瘤与软骨瘤的区别。

（1）软骨瘤

①软骨瘤好发于儿童，到成年后软骨瘤病变会停止生长。除非有病理性骨折，一般情况下软骨瘤是无痛的，中等大小，不会引起骨皮质内侧面的扇形生长，不会中断皮质骨，也不会引起软组织的肿胀。软骨瘤不影响皮质骨，除非它位于手和足的管状骨内。软骨肉瘤通常为中等大小，可引起骨皮质内侧面的贝壳样改变，不破坏骨皮质，不引起软组织肿胀。位于手的软骨性肿瘤几乎总是良性，因此在此部位只有在临床、影像学及组织学特征均表现为恶性改变时方可诊断为中心型软骨肉瘤。相反，躯干部位的软骨性肿瘤常为恶性，应高度怀疑为软骨肉瘤，除非经多年观察病变不发展，若怀疑时可行广泛切除。由于软骨瘤几乎均为良性，只有临床、影像学、病理学结果均提示为恶性时，才可考虑软骨肉瘤的诊断。与此相反，躯干部位多为软骨肉瘤，除非能证明是良性，比如病变界限清楚且数年未变，否则应考虑为软骨肉瘤。凡是怀疑为恶性者，均应行广泛切除。

②多发内生软骨瘤和内生软骨瘤病，肿瘤持续生长到成年，且肿瘤体积很大，增生活跃，常可恶变为软骨肉瘤。若成年人出现症状改变或有影像学改变，应行活检做病理检查，以确定是否发生恶变。

（2）关节滑膜软骨瘤

关节滑膜软骨瘤病的肿瘤围绕干骺端生长，呈分叶状，可迅速长大，填塞关节，侵犯关节囊、软组织，可广泛破坏骨关节。侵袭性关节滑膜软骨瘤病的大体病理表现和软骨肉瘤的非常相似，主要区别是软骨肉瘤很少侵入关节，而关节滑膜软骨瘤病常常位于关节内。

（3）成软骨细胞性骨肉瘤

首先是发病年龄，成软骨细胞性骨肉瘤发病年龄偏小，而软骨肉瘤一般发生在成人。鉴别关键在于组织检查，成软骨细胞性骨肉瘤即使可以存在软骨细胞，但一定伴有成骨细胞分化，且肿瘤细胞可有成骨表现。有时单纯依靠活检病理可能难以鉴别，因为成软骨细胞性骨肉瘤的治疗方案和软骨肉瘤的不一样，所以需先行化疗。这时可能需要切开活检，广泛取材，获得足够的病理标本。

（4）软骨黏液纤维瘤

软骨黏液纤维瘤与软骨肉瘤具有相似的大体表现，病理观察可发现中心小叶状细胞，有时难以区分其 Ⅰ、Ⅱ 级软骨肉瘤，这时需根据患者的发病特点、影像学表现及组织学仔细鉴别。

4.7 治疗方法

4.7.1 治疗前准备

软骨肉瘤应尽早治疗，虽然部分肿瘤生长缓慢，但高度恶性病例早期就可发生转移；低度恶性病例的恶性程度也可增加或去分化。治疗各种类型软骨肉瘤的唯一有效方法是行完整的外科切除。切除范围需要包括肿瘤假包膜和反应区，以及经过正常组织的广泛切除。边缘切除后的肿瘤复发危险性极大，软骨肉瘤复发后可能增加组织学上的恶性程度。

手术的设计及切除范围应取决于影像学检查（X线片、CT和MRI等）所提示的肿瘤侵犯范围。术前应进行局部穿刺或切开活检进行组织学分级，也可术中冰冻。由于活检标本可能不能反映整个软骨肉瘤的病理情况，因此若结果与临床症状及影像学检查结果不相符合，要重新取材或依据蜡块病理结果判断。活检时应注意彻底止血，以防止肿瘤在软组织中种植，再次手术时应切除原活检切口通路的所有组织。

对于普通型Ⅰ级软骨肉瘤，有文献认为可以采取相对保守的外科治疗方法。位于骨干内的Ⅰ级中心型软骨肉瘤可行广泛的病灶内切除，残腔采用苯酚、酒精、液氮等化学药物处理，可获得较满意的肢体功能结局，但仍有局部复发的危险。有文献报道，对于低度恶性软骨肉瘤，不完整切除的局部复发率也会高达70% ～ 80%。因为软骨肉瘤单纯刮除的手术成功率很低，所以不论病理级别，都不能采用这种手术方法。只可对处于软骨瘤和Ⅰ级软骨肉瘤间的病例行扩大的病灶内切除，并联合使用局部辅助治疗。最适合的治疗方法是行广泛或根治性切除。整段切除肿瘤后，要根据骨缺损的部位，采取不同的方法进行相应重建。

对于高度恶性的软骨肉瘤及去分化软骨肉瘤则更应采取广泛切除，有时甚至是根治性切除。但对于躯干的软骨肉瘤，则很难做到广泛切除，这种情况下通常患者预后不佳。随着近年来保肢技术的发展，大多数软骨肉瘤病例可以保留肢体。总体上，软骨肉瘤广泛切除的局部复发率可控制在10% ～ 15%。低度恶性的病例，即使复发后接受再次行广泛切除，仍有可能痊愈。对软组织侵犯明显的软骨肉瘤，尤其是Ⅲ级软骨肉瘤及去分化病例，常需要截肢方能控制。对于已经发生肺转移的病例，在允许的情况下进行转移瘤的切除，这样仍能延长患者的生命。

由于大多数软骨肉瘤是低度或中度恶性的肿瘤，确诊时肺转移并不常见，因此行广泛边界的外科切除将使大多数Ⅰ级普通软骨肉瘤及透明细胞软骨肉瘤等低度恶性病例得到痊愈。不同级别的软骨肉瘤预后不同，Ⅰ级软骨肉瘤生长缓慢，转移较少，5 年患者生存率达 90%，但若切除不充分可出现局部复发，肿瘤侵犯内脏及椎管可导致患者死亡；Ⅱ级软骨肉瘤虽然病程漫长，以及在组织学方面可能观察不到更多恶性的表现，但是也会发生早期转移，而且容易在局部复发，如果手术治疗及时且适当，治愈率可接近 60%；Ⅲ级软骨肉瘤预后最差，5 年患者生存率仅接近 40%。

软骨性肿瘤的病理级别是可以进级的，良性的内生软骨瘤或骨软骨瘤可以恶变为软骨肉瘤，低度恶性的可以进级为恶性程度更高的软骨肉瘤，甚至发生去分化改变，特别是在复发及转移病例中更常见。某学者治疗 21 例复发性骨盆软骨肉瘤，其中 8 例发生了恶性病理级别进级。在我们治疗的 33 例复发组随访病例中，发生了病理级别改变的有 15 例（45%）。一般认为，Ⅰ级软骨肉瘤即使多次复发也很少出现病理级别的改变，而且进展很缓慢；但Ⅱ级软骨肉瘤则可很快进展为Ⅲ级软骨肉瘤。

4.7.2　常见的治疗方法

①放疗、化疗

软骨肉瘤对放射治疗不敏感，放疗仅用于那些无法通过外科治疗达到广泛或根治性切除的病例，患者为缓解疼痛可以配合放疗。软骨肉瘤的化疗效果不稳定，仅在去分化软骨肉瘤中应用。化疗的效用尚不了解，原因是这些患者的年龄较大。软骨肉瘤的预后，主要与两个因素有关：组织学上的恶性程度及充分的切除术。化疗是否对去分化软骨肉瘤有效还存在争议。在我们治疗的去分化软骨肉瘤病例中，接受化疗的患者治疗效果并不明显，化疗未能阻止肿瘤转移的发生。Dickey 等总结化疗对去分化软骨肉瘤的作用，报道了从 1986—2000 年治疗的 42 例去分化软骨肉瘤病例，骨盆部位 12 例、股骨上端 16 例、肱骨上端 7 例、股骨下端 6 例、胫骨上端 1 例，男性 24 例、女性 18 例，平均年龄 66 岁（24～92.9 岁）。其中，单独接受手术切除 15 例，手术切除联合放疗 22 例，其余 5 例采用手术或活检加放、化疗。主要化疗药物包括阿霉素、顺铂、氨甲蝶呤。22 例手术联合化疗的病例中，除 1 例接受术后化疗外，其余患者均进行了新辅助化疗。在 39 例接受手术的患者中，18 例进行了截肢。对患者生存情况进行 Kaplan-Meier 分析，总体 5 年生存率为 7.1%，平均生存时间 7.5 个月。单纯手术组 5 年生存率为 11.8%，平均生存时间 6.4 个月；手术联合放疗组 5 年生存率 4%，平均生存时间 8.4 个月；两组之间生存率及生存时间无显著差异。这组患者的治疗结果与 1986 年以前的病例进行比较，治疗结果并无差异。这表明，尽管影像学检查、外科技术和辅助化疗的评估手段在近年来得到了很大的提高，但是去分化软骨肉瘤的预后仍然较差。一般认为，软骨肉瘤对化疗不敏感，但由于去分化软骨肉瘤中含有高度恶性的梭形细胞肉瘤（恶性纤维组织细胞瘤、骨肉瘤等），这些成分有可能对化疗敏感。研究表明，化疗可能对去分化软骨肉瘤患者有效，但病理标本的坏死率分析结果却显示去分化部分化疗后肿瘤坏死率＜90%。这种结果远比普通梭形细胞肉瘤的化疗反应差，反映出去分化软骨肉瘤的特殊生物学特性。Dickey 等人的研究结果表明，化疗不能有效控制去分化软骨肉瘤的远处转移和提高患者长期生存率，因此对这些患者采用化疗应当慎重。除了外科手术，去分化软骨肉瘤需要更有效的系统治疗方案，这可能包括生物治疗及分子靶向治疗。

因为间质性软骨肉瘤病例在无局部复发的情况下仍然有较高的转移率，所以部分研究将放疗联合化疗用于间质性软骨肉瘤，特别是不能进行根治性手术的病例，尽管这些治疗在本研究及其他报道中并没有显著、确定的疗效，但多数研究者认为，化疗及放疗联合化疗对部分间质性软骨肉瘤病例有效。

软骨肉瘤对化疗不敏感。一方面是与 MDR1 耐药基因及其产物 P-糖蛋白有关。在大多数软骨肉瘤中可以见到 MDR1 和 P-糖蛋白的表达，体外培养的软骨肉瘤细胞对阿霉素具有耐药性。另一个方面是软骨肉瘤具有大量的细胞外基质，阻止了抗肿瘤药物的进入。同时，软骨肉瘤一般生长较慢，这也导致其对化疗不敏感。

②分子靶向治疗

在内生软骨瘤、中央及周围型软骨肉瘤中，均存在甲状腺激素相关蛋白（PTHrP）信号通路活化，并随恶性程度的增加而升高的情况，说明该通路不仅影响正常生长软骨细胞的增殖，还会促进软骨肉瘤细胞生长。在成人骨骺闭合后，可以通过阻断 PTHrP 信号通路来抑制软骨肉瘤细胞的生长。由于 Bcl-2 是 PTHrP 的下游单位，并在周围及高级别中央型软骨肉瘤中表达，因此可以采用反义治疗的方法。但是 Bcl-2 具有抗凋亡作用，可能导致肿瘤耐药。阻断 Bcl-2 通路的试验药物已经应用于骨髓瘤的临床试验。在一项试验中，应用 PTHrP 的单克隆抗体可以下调 Bcl-2 的表达来诱导体外培养的软骨肉瘤细胞分化和凋亡。一项免疫组化研究结果显示，在软骨肉瘤中，血小板衍生生长因子受体（PDGF-R）呈阳性，表达程度与肿瘤恶性级别及患者生存率有关。如果该结果能被其他试验证实，则证明格列卫等靶向治疗药物可用于高度恶性软骨肉瘤的治疗。

③激素治疗

性激素，特别是雌激素通过影响骨骺生长板软骨细胞的增殖分化，对长骨的生长起重要调节作用。青春期生长高峰的开始及结束均受雌激素控制。在软骨肉瘤中，免疫组化试验发现雌激素受体呈阳性。另外，促进雌激素生物合成的芳香化酶在多数软骨肉瘤中均有表达。这些结果显示，软骨肉瘤可能和乳腺癌一样，对抗雌激素治疗敏感。

④抗血管生成治疗

基质金属蛋白酶 MMP1、MMP2、MMP9、MMP13 及 VEGF 在软骨肉瘤中均有表达，参与肿瘤局部侵犯和转移，并随恶性程度的增加而提高。MMP1 的 siRNA 治疗，在体外可以降低软骨肉瘤的侵袭性。血管内皮生长抑制剂也有可能减缓软骨肉瘤的生长和转移。有报道表明在软骨肉瘤动物模型上采用化疗联合抗血管生成治疗，导致肿瘤坏死及肿瘤血管减少。前列腺素 G/H 合酶 COX-2，可以促进血管生成，并在软骨肉瘤中表达，这提示用于结肠癌的选择性 COX-2 抑制剂可能对软骨肉瘤有效。

5　尤因肉瘤

5.1　定义

尤因肉瘤又称原发性神经外胚层肿瘤，是指具有不同程度神经外胚层特点的球形细胞肿瘤。在光镜或电镜下、免疫组化中，缺乏神经外胚层特征的肿瘤，则称为 Ewing 肉瘤；具有丰富神经外胚层特征的肿瘤，则称为原发性神经外胚层肿瘤。肿瘤细胞形态大小一致、排列致密，胞浆边界不清，核仁不明显，被纤维条索分隔，形成小叶或者条状形态。

5.2　流行病学

尤因肉瘤的发病率低于骨肉瘤、骨髓瘤、软骨肉瘤，占原发恶性骨肿瘤的 6% ～ 8%，不过它在儿童原发恶性骨肿瘤中排第二位。男性的 Ewing 肉瘤 / 原发性神经外胚层肿瘤发病率高于女性（1.4∶1），好发年龄低于 20 岁，一般为 10 ～ 20 岁。在 15 岁以下的患者中，尤因肉瘤是最常见的骨的肉瘤。此病在不同种族中发病率不一样，高加索人最好发，美国和非洲的黑人、东方人的发病率不高。尤因肉瘤的好发部位在股骨远端、胫骨近端，但也可侵及其他骨，包括骨盆、骶骨、肱骨和腓骨。

5.3　临床表现

尤因肉瘤最常见的临床症状是局部的疼痛。由于该肿瘤生长迅速，疼痛出现后几周即可触及肿块或出现局部肿胀，患者可能同时伴有发热、贫血、白细胞增多和血沉增快等表现，临床上容易被误诊为急性骨髓炎，不过很少会发生病理性骨折。

5.4　影像学表现

尤因肉瘤 X 线上的典型表现是长骨骨干骨髓腔呈斑片状溶骨性破坏，伴层状或葱皮状骨膜增生。肿瘤骨皮质厚薄不均，可看到长骨或扁平骨的骨干上边界不清的骨破坏灶、渗透性虫蚀样骨破坏。尤因肉瘤常表现为骨膨胀性破坏，可见到一个巨大的、边界不清的肿物。MRI 检查可以清晰地显示肿瘤浸润的范围，CT 检查有利于评价肿瘤在骨骼内的生长情况。

5.5　病理表现

尤因肉瘤细胞形态学表现并不一致，其中大多数是由有圆形细胞核的球形细胞组成。尤因肉瘤细胞大而不规则，核仁明显，染色体完好，但细胞质不清晰，细胞膜不清楚。在这种细胞的胞浆中可观察到含有过碘酸希夫染色（periodic acid-Schiff stain，PAS）染色呈阳性的糖原。部分肿瘤细胞可看到 Homer-Wright 环。肿瘤容易发生坏死，肿瘤细胞可浸润到血管周围。以前难以鉴别尤因肉瘤和恶性淋巴瘤，直到 1959 年有人在尤因肉瘤细胞中观察到糖原颗粒，才将其与恶性淋巴瘤区分。后来，PAS 染色的应用几乎可在所有尤因肉瘤中看到糖原成分，并以此获得了满意的病理检查结果。

尤因肉瘤除坏死区外仍有部分区域表现为糖原阴性。淋巴瘤和转移性神经母细胞瘤在糖原染色上均呈阴性。另外，唾液淀粉酶的处理也会导致糖原消失。PAS 核染色很少，一般都在胞浆内染色。即使是针吸活检小块标本或者细胞涂片标本，糖原染色都非常明显。可以使用福尔马林进行固定，如果使用 80% 的酒精，还可以固定碱性磷酸酶，染色效果更好。不建议使用强酸脱钙，因为其会影响糖原染色效果。因此，有时病理标本没有发现糖原成分并不能直接排除尤因肉瘤，需要考虑病理标本的处理是否有问题。

肿瘤细胞含有糖原成分并不一定是尤因肉瘤。比如，骨肉瘤中的去分化区域以及小细胞骨肉瘤也可以存在糖原成分，此时可以根据有无肿瘤性骨样基质以及通过测定碱性磷酸酶活性来鉴别。间充质软骨肉瘤的去分化区域也有细胞糖原阳性，但可通过在 X 线片和显微镜下观察有无软骨基质来鉴别。腺泡型或胚胎型横纹肌肉瘤的胞浆内有时也可以看见糖原成分，也容易将其与软组织尤因肉瘤混淆。

大多数尤因肉瘤的细胞膜上表达 CD99，但 CD99 并不是尤因肉瘤特异性的标志。另外，多数尤因肉瘤细胞中的波形蛋白（vimentin）、神经元特异性烯醇化酶常常表达阳性。角蛋白颗粒也可在部分尤因肉瘤 / 原发性神经外胚层肿瘤见到。

尤因肉瘤 / 原发性神经外胚层肿瘤的细胞基本为圆形或卵圆形，在胞浆可观察到糖原聚集物。在电镜下还可见到完整的细胞质和细胞内连接，并伴有神经分泌颗粒和微管。在电镜下观察肿瘤标本和组织培养的细胞，可以发现所有尤因肉瘤细胞内均含有糖原成分，这种现象在淋巴瘤和转移性神经母细胞瘤是没有的。

在电镜下观察，尤因肉瘤细胞呈多角形，胞浆少，有呈圆形或卵圆形的细胞核，有清楚、分布均匀的染色质，有清晰的核仁，细胞间可观察到连接结构。视野内还可观察到一种间质细胞，但其作用机制尚未研究清楚。

5.6　基因学

85% 的尤因肉瘤病例中都能观察到染色体 t（11；12）的改变，这是尤因肉瘤的特征。继发性染色体改变大多表现为染色体 8，9 和染色体臂 1q 的增加。染色体 t（11；12）的断裂点的分子克隆揭示了染色体臂 22q12 上 EWS 基因的 5′ 端和染色体 11q24 上 fli-1 基因的 3′ 端的融合，其中 fli-1 基因是 ETS 家族融合基因的一员。另外，还发现有 10% ～ 15% 的病例存在基因改变：t（21；22）（q22；q12），融合基因 EWS 迁移到染色体臂 21q22 上的 ETS 和 ERG 上。尤因肉瘤家族中不到 1% 的病例还存在其他基因改变：t（7；22）、t（17；2）、t（2；22）及 inv（22），它们分别提高了基因 EWS、ETS、ETV1、EIAF、FEV、ZSG 之间的融合。所以，几乎所有尤因肉瘤都会表达一定形式的融合基因 EWS/ETS。EWS/ETS 具有明显的致癌基因活性，而且有许多研究指出，EWS/ETS 及其他 EWS/ETS 化学绑定于 ETS 靶基因，作为异常迁移因素而发挥作用，可以在表达 EWS/FLI1 的细胞中找到许多上调基因，并观察到 EWS/ETS 蛋白。TGF-β Ⅱ型受体下调，TGF-β 在细胞中的减少，是尤因肉瘤家族逃避细胞程序性死亡的一个机制。尤因肉瘤家族第二常见的基因改变是 INK4a 的灭活，INK4a 是编码 CDKN2A 细胞周期的抑制因子。INK4a 的灭活导致 EWS/fli-1 抑癌蛋白的稳定表达。

染色体分析、反转录 · 聚合酶链反应（RT-PCR）、细胞间期杂交部位荧光染色、DNA 印迹法（Southern blotting）都是尤因肉瘤基因诊断的方法，最好同时联合使用一种以上的方法进行检测，以避免误差。外周血和骨髓的融合拷贝检测对微小残留的病灶比较敏感，但其临床意义还有待进一步明确。

5.7　外周循环中尤因肉瘤细胞的分子探测

RT-PCR 用于在尤因肉瘤上探测骨与软组织肿瘤患者的循环肿瘤细胞。尤因肉瘤是儿童第二大常见的原发骨肿瘤。尽管全身化疗提高了总生存率，但长期生存率仍限制在 50% ～ 60% 之间。转移灶的存在与否是影响预后的关键因素。尤因肉瘤好发的转移部位是肺、骨髓，并且都是血源性传播，转移灶的检查主要是肺和骨的 CT 等影像学表现以及骨髓的细胞学和组织学分析。由于尤因肉瘤细胞缺乏特异性标志，所以骨髓污染有时难以检测到，这意味着容易忽略部分转移灶的存在。因此，通过外周血和骨髓的肿瘤细胞的敏感探测对于尤因肉瘤的分期和随访非常重要。

近年来，尤因肉瘤特征性染色体易位 t（11；22）（q24；q12）的克隆已成为尤因肉瘤新的肿瘤标志，这种染色体的畸变导致了 22 号染色体的 EWS 基因与 11 号染色体的 fli-1 基因融合。部分尤因肉瘤的 22 号和 21 号染色体重排，能够引起 EWS 基因与 ERG 基因融合。RT-PCR 技术可以探测到这些融合基因编码融合转录。95% 以上的尤因肉瘤与 EWS/fli-1 或 EWS/ERG 融合转录有关。另外，约 90% 的尤因肉瘤和 PNET 肿瘤有 t（11；22）（q24；q12）基因易位，造成 EWS/fli-1 或 EWS/ERG 融合转录。因此，这种用于诊断和监测尤因肉瘤残余病灶的融合转录，可作为一种特异的和高度敏感的核酸肿瘤标志。取患者的外周血或骨髓进行检测，若能探测到 EWS/fli-1 RNA，则提示肿瘤的亚显微沉积或隐伏的肿瘤细胞。

5.8 诊断与鉴别诊断

5.8.1 尤因肉瘤的诊断

尤因肉瘤放射学表现多样，可能被误诊为其他疾病。葱皮样改变是尤因肉瘤的典型特征，但不是所有的尤因肉瘤都会有此表现，而且骨髓炎、嗜酸性肉芽肿和骨肉瘤也可能表现为葱皮样改变，这只是反应性骨膜反应的表现。尤因肉瘤有时也可以表现出日光放射线征象和 Codman 三角。新生骨由骨膜产生，而且被快速生长的肿块顶离骨皮质。Codman 三角中肿块从葱皮样分层的中心部分侵出，仅离开 Codman 三角的底边。日光放射线征象的中心部分由针状新骨充填并垂直向骨干放射。髓腔内溶骨性破坏是尤因肉瘤的常见表现，骨质可呈现鼠蚀样改变，从而可与骨肉瘤鉴别。少部分尤因肉瘤以成骨为主要表现，这也导致大量反应骨形成。CT 及 MRI 扫描检查对于尤因肉瘤的诊断非常关键，可以发现大的与骨相连的软组织肿块，这个表现在 X 线片中不易被发现。特殊部位的尤因肉瘤，如骨盆尤因肉瘤的骨膜反应常无放射学证据，此时软组织在诊断中变得更为重要。化验室检查显示白细胞升高、血沉增加，同时伴有发热、局部肿胀疼痛表现，这些表现容易让临床医师将其误诊为骨髓炎。

5.8.2　尤因肉瘤与其他疾病的诊断

尤因肉瘤在影像学上的表现，使其有时很难与骨梅毒、骨嗜酸性肉芽肿、骨肉瘤、骨髓炎等疾病区分开来，最终可能需要病理诊断进行明确。组织学上，尤因肉瘤有时候容易和未分化的神经母细胞瘤混淆。神经母细胞瘤在成人中很少见，常发生在 5 岁以下儿童，经常有颅骨转移灶、眼球突出的表现，病变位置一般在长骨干骺端。另外，神经母细胞瘤糖原表达阴性，故可通过 PAS 染色进行鉴别。而且，尿中儿茶酚胺水平升高是神经母细胞瘤的特征。电镜下神经母细胞瘤可观察到神经颗粒和神经纤维。小圆细胞肉瘤和间充质软骨肉瘤可以观察到小圆细胞，可以通过有无骨基质和软骨基质成分进行鉴别。

尤因肉瘤早期容易扩散，容易转移至肺和其他骨，且转移范围广。尤因肉瘤容易侵及骨髓，这一特点在其他肉瘤中不常见。Meyers 等发现，侵及骨髓的尤因肉瘤患者是没有幸存的，表明骨髓侵袭是尤因肉瘤不良预后的高危因素。尤因肉瘤标准分期研究需要进行活组织检查。

5.9　治疗方法

5.9.1　放疗

尤因肉瘤的治疗仍然存在很大的争议，放疗、化疗、手术或联合治疗都是治疗尤因肉瘤的方法。既往最常应用放疗。肿瘤对放疗敏感，这已经被 Ewing 和其他学者证实。然而，尤因肉瘤早期就存在微转移灶，单纯行放疗，患者的生存率不高于 10%。许多学者强烈反对手术治疗尤因肉瘤，因为为了完全切除病灶，常常直接截肢，手术结果令人不满意。

放疗应用于肿瘤局部的控制率为 60% ～ 90%。放疗在尤因肉瘤治疗方面的应用已发展很长时间，早期仪器的限制导致放疗受到阻碍。随着诊疗技术的发展，CT 和 MRI 能更准确地描绘肿物，给放疗提供更好的视野，这使得放疗有所发展，但放疗的效果仍不乐观。某学者报告的尤因肉瘤局部控制达三年的只有76%。研究报道，仅 77% 局部控制达到五年。有学者发现，26 例肿瘤患者有 50% 出现复发，这表明放疗仍有较大局限性。

许多因素都影响放疗的效果。首要影响因素是肿瘤的大小，相比于小肿瘤，在大肿瘤内更有可能存在耐照射的细胞群。肿瘤的发生部位也影响放疗效果，骨盆肿瘤和脊柱肿瘤放疗后的复发率比四肢肿瘤更高。

5.9.2　化疗

化疗是治疗尤因肉瘤的重要手段。相比不化疗的患者，接受化疗的患者的总体局部复发率较低。某学者发现对化疗反应好的患者，其局部控制率高于对化疗反应差的患者。在这项研究中，肿瘤小于 8 cm 且对化疗有阳性反应的患者，在进行小剂量放疗后，局部控制率达到 90%；肿瘤大于 8 cm 且对化疗有阳性反应的患者，在进行大剂量放疗后，局部控制率为 52%。而对化疗反应差的患者，虽然也进行大剂量放疗，但最终局部控制率仅有 17%。

5.9.3 手术

手术最大的临床意义，是可去除大肿瘤内存在的耐放疗及化疗的细胞群。另外，有学者认为，经过放疗的患者有继发骨肉瘤的危险，放疗的剂量越大，时间越长，恶变的危险性越高。

许多临床医师反对手术，他们认为手术是有创的、具有破坏性的，而放疗是无创且保肢的，所以他们更倾向于放疗。然而，随着手术重建器械的显著发展，保肢手术后肢体功能已明显改善，这些观点已不完全适用。手术的风险越来越低，使用现代外科器械进行骨缺损部位重建，比如肋骨、锁骨和腓骨，已经获得了良好的术后功能。另外，放疗也难以避免损害正常组织，可能产生一系列功能障碍，放疗还伴有一系列并发症，比如关节挛缩、脉管炎、神经病变、生长平台停滞、皮肤萎缩和脱落、肌肉纤维化、肢体增长不足、骨坏死和病理性骨折。

相对于功能的影响，肿瘤学结果对选择手术还是放疗的更为重要。尽管现在仍没有定论，但一些研究已显示手术的局部控制率高于放疗的。Bacci 等发现，单纯手术或手术加放疗的局部复发率仅 8%，远远低于单纯行放疗的局部复发率（36%）。有学者报道，手术加放疗的复发率为 4%，单纯放疗的局部复发率为 15%，单纯手术的复发率为 4%。但是这些研究都不是随机临床试验，手术切除的病例大多是较小的和远端的肿瘤，因此结论有明显偏倚。

中心部位的大的尤因肉瘤预后效果普遍较差，因为这些部位难以划定手术部位，且并发症发生率高，因此不建议行手术治疗，建议行放疗。但肿瘤与重要器官毗邻，即使放疗治愈仍然非常困难，且放疗后这些肿瘤局部复发率高。

目前，尚没有最佳的治疗方法可适于所有尤因肉瘤患者。理论上，手术可降低局部复发率，但并不适用于所有患者，病变必须有可切除的明确的边界，能够设计良好的手术范围，因此必须认真选择适合患者的手术设计。手术和放疗联合使用有利于降低高危患者的复发率，但放疗后进行手术容易出现伤口并发症。无法接受手术切除的患者，可以选择进行放疗。经过放疗和诱导化疗后，病变可能缩小并符合手术条件。

随着现代治疗技术的发展，Ewing 肉瘤 / 原发性神经外胚层肿瘤的生存率已达到 41%，预后较前已有了很大提高。肿瘤的分期、解剖部位、大小都是重要的预后因素。早期转移或骨盆肿瘤提示预后不良。另外，EWS/ETS 融合，EWS 及其相邻基因之间不同片段的融合导致不同程度的异常蛋白升高，这也会影响肿瘤的预后。那些具有 EWS/fli-1 基因融合的局部肿瘤中，相比于具有更广泛、更少见的融合类型的肿瘤，即最常见的 I 型基因融合预后更好。

6　骨转移瘤

6.1　定义及流行病学

骨转移是成年人骨破坏最常见的原因。大约一半的癌症患者会发生骨转移。乳腺、肺、肾、前列腺、肝、甲状腺等是常见的原发癌症部位。癌症转移的细胞异常迅速生长，可以导致患者出现骨痛、骨折、高钙血症、贫血和神经压迫等症状。不同癌症出现骨转移的概率并不一致，乳腺癌和前列腺癌出现骨转移的概率通常为 65% ～ 75%，多发性骨髓瘤为 70% ～ 95%，甲状腺癌为 60%，肺癌为 30% ～ 40%，黑色素瘤为 14% ～ 45%，肾癌为 20% ～ 25%。大多数转移瘤呈现溶骨性改变，但个别肿瘤，比如前列腺癌可以表现为成骨性改变。骨科医生需要对很多骨转移患者进行处理。若病变骨未骨折，建议给予预防性处理使其不发生骨折；若病变骨已发生骨折，建议行适当的固定。骨转移瘤患者的数量相比于原发性骨肿瘤的要多很多，因此骨科医生应当熟悉骨转移性肿瘤的诊疗原则。

脊柱、骶骨、骨盆、肋骨、四肢的近端都是骨转移瘤常发生的部位，膝和肘以外的部位不常见。肺转移容易侵及肢体远端，前列腺癌和乳腺癌很少发生肢体远端的转移。脊柱静脉系统在骨转移中非常关键。乳腺癌、肺癌、前列腺癌、肾癌、甲状腺癌都可以直接引流到脊柱静脉系统，再通过该系统与椎体、骨盆、肋骨、头颅骨和肢体近端相通。

6.2　骨转移瘤致溶骨性破坏的分子基础

肿瘤细胞介导破骨细胞异常激活，这是癌症患者骨骼被破坏的主要分子机制。肿瘤细胞能刺激机体生成 PTHrP 产生高钙血症，也能直接刺激局部骨微环境中破骨细胞生成和激活。破骨细胞是在溶骨性骨吸收过程中的主要效应细胞。破骨细胞的起源是单核–巨噬细胞系统造血细胞。破骨细胞被激活后可以产生溶骨作用，然后介导细胞凋亡的最终过程。

介导破骨细胞的生成以不同细胞因子为主导，并与其他相关因子相互作用，这些病理过程导致了骨转移瘤的溶骨性损害。参与溶骨的细胞能够分泌能溶解骨基质的蛋白酶类，同时分泌具有释放骨骼矿物质并进入细胞外间隙作用的酸类物质，从而完成溶骨过程。一些溶骨性骨吸收调节因子，如甲状旁腺激素、前列腺素，可以调控破骨细胞分泌氢离子。一类质子泵参与了破骨细胞分泌酸的酸化过程，另一类空泡型质子泵类似肾脏的氢离子 ATP 酶，通过非浓度依赖性的方式转运质子，参与溶骨性骨吸收的过程。碳酸酐酶等酶类的酶促反应为质子泵提供了质子。破骨细胞高水平表达水解酶、基质金属蛋白酶（matrix metalloproteinase，MMP）和胶原酶共同作用从而降解胶原基质。

骨转移瘤的患者中，肿瘤细胞分泌多种细胞因子，进一步刺激病理状态下的破骨细胞生成，最终导致溶骨性骨骼破坏。溶骨性骨吸收过程，可以使骨基质进一步释放多种刺激肿瘤细胞增殖的生长因子。肿瘤细胞与破骨细胞间相互作用，最终导致了肿瘤细胞刺激破骨细胞生成和异常性骨吸收增强，而增强的骨吸收过程又进一步释放促进肿瘤生长的各种细胞因子，形成了恶性循环。

6.3 临床表现

疼痛是骨转移瘤患者最常见的表现，可以表现为局部性的疼痛或者是弥散性的疼痛。如果病变位于长骨上，疼痛往往局限于病变的部位；如果病变位于骨盆或者脊柱、骶骨上，疼痛就不仅仅是局限于病变的部位，还可同时出现神经压迫症状及其他表现，导致较难明确病变部位。恶性骨肿瘤的疼痛一般是静息痛，表现为不能耐受负重，关节活动受限。刚开始时疼痛呈间断性，逐渐加重后可变为持续性的，并常常伴有夜间疼痛。当这种破坏性的骨病变位于股骨等负重骨上时，患者主要表现为行走时疼痛。如果负重时患者出现严重的疼痛，且在 X 线片上可观察到较大的溶骨性骨破坏时，应该考虑到可能很快发生溶骨性的骨折。可能出现骨折的最主要症状之一就是负重时疼痛，比如在行走时下肢发生疼痛。出现症状时往往骨质破坏已经超过 50%。完全溶骨性破坏非常容易发生骨折，而完全成骨性则很少发生骨折，混合性的则很难确定。

实际上，所有的骨转移瘤患者的平均生存期为 6 ～ 48 个月，最终死亡一般都是原发病导致的。对骨转移瘤患者而言，治疗的主要目的是控制疼痛，以及保持肢体功能。然而，不同患者的预后差异很大。一般而言，前列腺癌、肾癌、甲状腺癌和乳腺癌患者的生存期相对较长，因而对生活治疗的期望比较高，而肺癌和肝癌患者的一般生存期低于 1 年，因而对生活治疗的期望较低。

6.4 诊断

如果老年患者出现多发性骨破坏，首先需要考虑骨转移性病变，当然也不排除多发性骨髓瘤及甲状旁腺功能亢进等疾患。血液学及全身骨扫描等检查是必需的。如果明确患者患有骨转移疾病，需要对患者即将发生的骨折或者已经发生的病理性骨折进行评估和治疗。有癌症病史的患者有可能发生单骨转移、多骨转移或者骨和内脏转移。如果病变范围广，出现弥漫性的骨和内脏转移，即使没有组织学诊断，医师也应该想到是骨转移瘤，并且按计划给予进一步诊断与治疗。如果患者有癌症病史，但是术后没有局部复发，表现为孤立骨病变，就不能假定该病是原发瘤转移。这种情况应该先行活检以明确诊断。孤立骨病变的患者有可能患有原发性骨肿瘤，应该仔细评估和给予活检。

成年人（超过40岁）的骨转移瘤有可能是单个的骨破坏而没有癌症病史。尽管骨转移在成年人中并不多见，但是在诊断时应考虑这种可能性。全身检查，包括彻底的体格检查、B超、骨扫描及化验检查等，在这种情况下是必要的。在没有足够的依据时，就不能随意推测任何破坏性的病变都是转移性的；在没有活检病理结果前不应该直接给予手术固定，这可能会引起不正确的治疗并造成严重后果。尽管大部分患者是转移瘤，行髓内针固定是合适的，但少部分患者可能是肉瘤，直接行髓内针会造成广泛的肿瘤污染，导致本来可以保留肢体的患者最后必须截肢。

骨转移瘤的确诊方法主要是穿刺活检取标本行病理检查。穿刺针活检或者在CT引导下行细针穿刺活检，这样确诊率高，并且容易操作。穿刺点的选择也非常重要。如果是单发病变，穿刺点需要考虑放在随后的手术切口线上，一旦病变是恶性肿瘤，可以在手术时同时切除穿刺点，不至于造成肿瘤污染伤口。此外，骨扫描可以明确骨转移病变的范围，X线片有助于发现容易穿刺的部位。CT检查可以协助骨盆穿刺时设计穿刺的部位和进针路线，因为穿刺针必须通过皮质骨的反应区到达病变的核心区，CT透视结果可以帮助更好地设计手术方案。另外，穿刺应该避免将穿刺针穿入反应区的硬化骨，因为那个部位可能没有肿瘤细胞。

6.5　治疗

骶骨转移瘤并不十分常见，但治疗有较大的困难。骶骨转移瘤的对症治疗，主要是对转移部位肿瘤进行放疗以缓解症状，同时针对原发灶进行化疗以及免疫治疗。神经受压所致的大小便功能以及下肢功能的异常，都是对症治疗的内容。部分患者接受放疗或化疗等保守治疗手段可以改善症状，但是对于一些严重疼痛以及明显神经受压的患者，保守治疗难以提高他们的活动或者大小便功能异常的情况，特别是生存期相对比较长的患者，需要进行手术治疗。多数骶骨转移瘤的治疗是姑息性手术，手术的目的是缓解患者的症状、改善患者的生活质量。骶骨周围重要的组织和结构比较多，解剖结构复杂，并且血供丰富，因此，对骶骨转移瘤的手术的原则是简单有效。骶骨转移瘤的手术以刮除为主，一般不进行根治性或者广泛切除，除非是部分预后相对比较好的肿瘤。

骶骨周围血供丰富，骶骨转移瘤异常增生的血管使手术的风险比其他位置肿瘤的手术风险要高得多。骶骨转移瘤的手术方式非常复杂，术后需要对患者进行严密观察，护理也需要丰富的经验。术前应该充分评估患者的一般情况，严格掌握好适应证。多数转移瘤患者的一般情况并不好，术前要对患者进行多方面的检查，包括心肺功能、肝肾功能、电解质情况等，及时纠正负平衡，纠正贫血等不利手术恢复的因素。肾癌、肝癌、肺癌等肿瘤，血供比较丰富，如果肿瘤体积较大，为减少术中出血，应该常规进行术前栓塞或者前路阻断供血血管。

既往并没有明确的文献说明骶骨转移瘤手术治疗的适应证。在明确外科治疗目的的情况下，对骶骨转移瘤的适应证以及手术方式的选择要做到个体化。骶骨转移瘤外科治疗的目的有以下几种：①解除肿瘤对神经的压迫，减轻剧烈疼痛，提高生存质量，减少使用镇痛药物；②解除肿瘤对神经的压迫，恢复神经功能，比如大小便功能、四肢功能；③减轻病灶引起的机械性不稳定，重建骶髂关节周围的稳定性，缓解活动引起的疼痛，改善下肢功能，恢复生活自理能力；④病理明确诊断，分析患者的病变，为后续治疗提供依据。转移瘤的外科手术治疗无法延长患者的生存时间，因此骶骨转移瘤的外科手术治疗，至少不应增加患者的痛苦。目前，骶骨转移瘤的外科手术仍然面临许多问题，其中最核心的问题是如何综合判断患者的手术适应证及手术时机。只有充分评估患者的全身状况，综合评定肿瘤的性质、转移灶的数量、病变的范围，方能制订良好的治疗方案。

骶骨周围毗邻的重要组织和结构较多，局部解剖关系复杂，肿瘤血供比较丰富，术前一定要充分认识到手术的风险，特别是出血风险，术前的周密准备对手术成功至关重要。除了常规的术前准备，术前还要进行肠道准备和控制出血的准备。对出血的控制：骶骨转移瘤的手术治疗出血量非常大，一般在 3000～5000 mL，如果肿瘤血供丰富、体积比较大，出血量甚至可以达 10000～20000 mL。出血量大于 4000～5000 mL 时，术中就可能出现凝血功能的异常，主要表现为创面大量渗血，血液明显稀释，凝血速度减慢。骶骨周围的血管非常多，骶骨前方又是比较疏松的组织，无法将血肿局限于切口周围，渗出的血液可能沿腹膜后的间隙向周围延伸，为了避免出现致命性的出血，术中就要及时补充血浆以及凝血因子。因此术前要准备充足的血源，除了常规的红细胞、血浆，血小板以及相应的凝血因子也必须充分准备。除了血源准备，控制出血的有效手段还包括术前进行肿瘤血管栓塞。栓塞应该在手术的当天或者前一天进行。如果栓塞过早，肿瘤周围血管增生会导致栓塞失效。栓塞常见的并发症包括供血区域的疼痛以及术后发热，需要对症处理。另外，临时血管阻断术，包括术前放置腹主动脉球囊阻断，以及术中临时阻断腹主动脉的同时进行髂内动脉结扎，这是最有效的控制出血的手段。常规手段应该在骶骨转移瘤手术前放置球囊阻断腹主动脉血流，这样能够明显地控制手术当中的出血，从而降低术中大出血的危险。前侧入路可以进行腹主动脉临时阻断以及髂内动脉结扎，也可以有效地控制出血。另外，还可以对以一侧髂内动脉供血为主的骶骨肿瘤单纯进行髂内动脉结扎来减少出血量。

单纯前侧入路、单纯后侧入路和前后侧联合入路都是骶骨肿瘤手术常用的入路方式。转移瘤的外科手术以刮除为主，因此最常用的血管阻断术的手术方式是后侧入路。有时候为了更好地控制出血，可以采取前后侧联合入路从而提高骶骨截除术的安全性。如果能使用栓塞技术和腹主动脉阻断技术，可以大大减少手术出血，因此现在已经很少使用前侧入路的血管阻断术。

控制出血是骶骨手术中的重要步骤。控制出血才能有清晰的手术野，才能比较彻底地切除肿瘤，才能保护神经根以及进行神经松解术。如果同时进行前路的血管阻断术，进行阻断的时机应该选择在将骶骨后侧的软组织分开之后进入肿瘤之前。在分离骶骨后侧的软组织过程中要注意沿组织的解剖间隙进行，尽量避免出血。清除骶骨肿瘤过程要避免不必要的重复步骤，使手术快速有效。手术中要避免出现血容量快速降低的现象，同时要和麻醉医师相互协作。肿瘤清除后形成的残腔，可以采用适当的填充物填塞，这样不但可以填充肿瘤切除术后形成的残腔，也能够有效地控制出血。缝合过程要抓紧时间，同时对切除肿瘤的部位进行加压止血。术后要注意检查电解质、血常规、凝血功能等，及时纠正贫血以及凝血功能的异常。

骶骨转移瘤容易侵犯的神经包括坐骨神经和阴部内神经。S1 支配小腿后群肌，S2 主要支配大腿后群肌，S2 ～ S4 组成阴部内神经，和交感、副交感神经纤维共同支配膀胱和直肠括约肌功能及性功能。绝大部分骶骨转移瘤都会侵犯 S1 和 S2，并且采取的手术方案多为肿瘤刮除术，因此术中要尽量谨慎操作，最大程度保留患者的神经完整性。S1 神经保留是保持正常步态的关键，保留仅仅单侧 S1 和 S2 神经会导致仅有少部分患者能保留正常的肠道功能和膀胱功能；保留双侧 S1 和 S2 神经则可使大部分患者能保留正常的肠道功能和膀胱功能；单侧 S1 ～ S3 神经切除后患者同侧会阴部感觉麻木，但不影响性功能。骶骨转移瘤的外科手术治疗目的一般为对症治疗和姑息治疗，在手术条件允许的情况下，应该尽量保留患者的神经功能，以提高患者的生存质量。根据具体情况，在不影响肿瘤较为彻底切除的条件下，应该尽可能保留双侧 S1、S2 及至少一侧 S3 神经根，同时配合适当的功能锻炼，可以最大限度保留行走、大小便及性功能。

骶骨是骶髂关节的重要组成部分，负责将躯体部分的重量向下肢传导，骶髂关节受到损伤，将严重影响脊柱的稳定性。切除不同阶段的骶骨肿瘤后对骶髂关节的稳定性有不同程度的影响，骶骨肿瘤切除后是否进行骶骨重建一直存在争论。是否行重建手术取决于髂骨翼的切除范围及患者的患病情况，应避免出现严重并发症，使患者更快康复。全骶骨或次全骶骨切除后如果不进行骶骨重建，只能依靠骶骨和骨盆之间、骶骨和脊柱之间的韧带组织、残留的关节以及术后形成的瘢痕组织维持稳定性，因此患者需要长时间卧床。近年来，随着脊柱内固定器械的快速发展，许多医生对行全骶骨切除术后的患者实施内固定手术，以达到重建脊柱骶骨稳定性的目的。由于 S2 神经参与构成骶髂关节的大部分，S2 及以上水平切除的患者应该进行辅助固定以加强骨盆环的稳定性。

总之，骶骨肿瘤邻近部位解剖结构复杂，早期症状隐匿，容易被误诊或漏诊，确诊时肿瘤已经很大，会给手术带来困难。早期及时的诊断是彻底切除骶骨肿瘤的重要条件，外科治疗效果较满意，是首选的治疗方法。为了明显减少术中出血、提高手术的安全性，可以实施前路髂内动脉结扎、暂时阻断腹主动脉或术前数字减影血管造影（DSA）介入栓塞。尽可能保留 S1 ～ S3 神经对于保留患者功能、提高术后生活质量非常重要。骶骨重建骨盆稳定性，可使患者更快康复。辅助放疗、化疗可减少复发，提高疗效。

第2部分　高位骶骨恶性肿瘤外科治疗结局研究

1　研究背景与意义

1.1　全骶骨切除术治疗高位骶骨恶性肿瘤

临床上以脊索瘤最多见，其次为骨巨细胞瘤，骶骨肿瘤比较少见。其中原发高度恶性骨肿瘤更为少见，主要包括骨肉瘤、软骨肉瘤、尤因肉瘤等。脊索瘤是低度恶性肿瘤，如果为了保留骶神经的功能而采取瘤内手术，则难以避免术后的高复发率，因此文献报道一般采取整块切除手术，虽然牺牲了一部分骶神经的功能，但是相比瘤内手术，复发率能明显降低。而对于骶骨的高度恶性肿瘤，如骨肉瘤、软骨肉瘤、尤因肉瘤等，为了降低局部复发率，达到治愈的结果，必须行广泛性切除手术。全骶骨切除术的绝对适应证是累及 S2 以上神经的脊索瘤和原发高度恶性骨肿瘤；相对适应证是累及全骶骨的骨巨细胞瘤及神经源性肿瘤。

关于手术入路的问题，对于高位骶骨肿瘤，为充分暴露病灶，多数文献报道采取前后路联合的手术方式。但是，前后路联合的手术入路因为需要更换体位，手术时间较长，而且前路手术有发生局部种植转移的风险，因此，有学者对高位骶骨肿块向前突出较小的肿块进行了单纯后路全骶骨切除的手术，同样获得良好的外科边界及肿瘤学预后。

对于全骶骨切除术，控制术中出血非常重要。高位骶骨肿瘤的体积巨大，局部解剖结构复杂，主要的血管供应包括双侧髂内动脉、骶正中动脉及其与腹主动脉和髂外动脉的侧支循环。术中大量出血，不仅容易导致术野暴露不清，从而难以保证良好的外科边界，而且也容易发生失血性休克，提高患者围手术期的死亡率、术中及术后并发症的发生率，还会提高肿瘤局部复发率。控制骶骨肿瘤手术出血的方法包括腹主动脉球囊阻断、术前血管栓塞和术中前路结扎髂内动脉及临时阻断腹主动脉。其中，腹主动脉球囊阻断可以有效减少术中出血量，同时，相较其他血管阻断方式而言对患者的损伤更小，术后并发症发生率更低，提高了手术的安全性。

实施全骶骨切除术后，骨盆环被破坏，腰椎和骨盆完全分离，如果不进行重建，患者需要长期卧床，依靠手术瘢痕的形成来限制脊柱的下沉。如果术中进行重建，患者可以尽早恢复行走功能，减少术后卧床并发症，但是要注意重建会增加伤口感染的风险。文献报道的骶髂关节重建方式，基本是采用不同的钢棒、钢板和螺钉的组合，或者结合植骨的方法。

全骶骨切除术常见的术后并发症，包括伤口并发症、脑脊液漏、肠道损伤、下肢深静脉血栓、内固定失败以及神经功能损伤等。处理伤口并发症视情况而定，部分患者需行手术引流、清创和Ⅱ期伤口闭合处理。脑脊液漏一般可通过抬高床尾、使用抗生素等治疗手段处理。如果术中发现肠壁部分损伤但未完全穿透肠壁，可以术中行肠壁修补；如果已经穿破肠壁，则应行结肠造瘘手术。实施全骶骨切除术后，由于手术创伤大，患者卧床时间较长，形成下肢深静脉血栓的风险较高，可通过穿抗栓袜、预防性使用抗凝药物等手段降低其发生的风险。如果出现内固定物周围感染，应及时将内固定物取出，行旷置处理；如果出现内固定物松动、断裂，需综合考虑患者的活动功能、疼痛程度、经济条件等，再决定是否行内固定翻修手术。

既往文献报道的全骶骨切除术后患者复发率在 8.0% ～ 57.1% 之间。2000 年，Wuisman 等报道的 9 例全骶骨切除术后患者中 3 例死于肿瘤的复发与转移，1 例出现孤立肺转移的骨巨细胞瘤，患者接受手术处理病灶后在随访期间（90 个月）无瘤生存，另外 5 例在随访期间（范围 30 ～ 120 个月，平均 73 个月）无复发证据。2000 年，Miles 等报道了 25 例全骶骨切除术后患者，平均随访时间 16 个月（范围 10 天～ 44 个月），出现局部复发 2 例，死于肺转移 1 例。2003 年，Doita 等报道了 3 例全骶骨切除术后患者，其中 1 例死于肿瘤的复发。2005 年，Dickey 等报道了 5 例全骶骨切除术后患者，平均随访时间 18 个月，其中 2 例死于肿瘤的复发与转移。2008 年，刘世清等报道了 7 例全骶骨切除术后患者，术后随访 6 ～ 36 个月，其中 4 例死于肿瘤的复发或转移。2014 年，孙伟等报道了 5 例全骶骨切除术后患者，其中出现局部复发 1 例，随访期间带瘤生存。由于高位骶骨恶性肿瘤的低发病率以及手术的高难度，既往文献报道的全骶骨切除术的例数都比较少，因此，需要更多病例的数据以获得更加准确的结论。

1.2 全骶骨切除术后患者的神经功能评估

全骶骨切除术在术中会切除双侧 S1 及以下神经，因此无可避免地会丧失双侧 S1 及以下神经的功能，造成严重的下肢运动功能、大小便功能及性功能的损伤。

20 世纪 70 年代，Gunterberg 等对骶骨肿瘤切除术后的神经功能损伤进行研究，包括大小便功能和性功能的研究，这被认为是这一领域的第一次系统研究。他们通过测量患者的直肠容积和压力、肛门内括约肌区压力和肛门外括约肌肌电活动，研究了 3 例切除了双侧骶神经和 4 例切除了单侧骶神经的患者的肛门直肠功能。他们发现，丧失双侧骶神经会造成严重的大便失禁或便秘，直肠扩张的感觉同样受到了损害，肛门内括约肌压力正常但是肛门外括约肌的功能丧失；仅保留双侧 S2 以上神经时，患者无法对通过直肠的内容物进行准确鉴别；而丧失单侧骶神经患者的肛门直肠功能无明显损害。为了评价膀胱功能，他们对 5 例切除了双侧骶神经的患者和 4 例切除了单侧骶神经的患者进行了研究，研究内容主要有临床评价、膀胱计量学和膀胱镜检查，包括不同刺激下的膀胱和尿道敏感性测试。他们发现，研究人员无法观察到仅保留双侧 S2 及以上神经的患者的逼尿肌的活动性收缩，从而认为 S2 神经无法单独促成逼尿肌反射。还发现切除双侧 S3 及以下骶神经后患者膀胱黏膜痛觉消失，而保留 S3 神经的患者则膀胱黏膜痛觉正常。仅切除单侧骶神经的患者，膀胱功能基本正常，但是会丧失切除神经一侧膀胱黏膜的痛觉和温觉。为了评估性功能，他们研究了 9 例骶骨肿瘤根治性切除的患者（5 例双侧骶神经切除和 4 例单侧骶神经切除）。对男性患者，他们测量了射精期间从外尿道和肛门括约肌之间的肌电活动，认为阴茎的感觉是由 S2 神经支配的。对女性患者，他们进行了性生活史的询问和敏感性测试，发现 2 例切除了双侧 S3 至 S5 神经的女性患者性功能未受明显损害。单侧骶神经完全切除的患者具备接近正常的性功能，只是患侧感觉会丧失。1986 年，Andreoli 等对 1 例切除了双侧 S2 及以下神经的患者和 1 例切除了单侧 S2 及以下神经的患者进行研究，认为至少保留 1 根 S2 神经就足以维持患者的大小便控制能力而不至于大小便失禁。1994 年，Fujimura 等研究 8 例骶骨肿瘤根治性切除双侧骶神经的患者，对患者的下肢运动功能和感觉、大小便功能、性功能以及其他日常生活能力进行了评估，认为保留 L5 及以上神经对于患者维持行走能力是必需的；保留 S2 及以上神经能够让患者保留一定的大小便功能和性功能，以具备基本的日常生活能力；而保留双侧 S3 及以上神经的患者，其下肢运动功能和感觉、大小便功能、性功能及其他日常生活能力几乎不受影响。

早期的这些研究表明，分析骶神经切除的范围和神经功能损伤之间的联系，具有非常积极的意义，但之前的研究都属于个案分析或小样本的研究，所以得出的结论可能会有偏倚。近些年来的一些文献样本量更大一些，得出的结论也更具准确性。2002 年、2005 年、2006 年、2009 年先后有 4 篇文章报道了 53 例、11 例、16 例、17 例骶骨肿瘤根治性切除后的神经功能结果，得出的结论与之前文献的报道基本一致，证实了前人研究的准确性。

然而，长期以来，骶骨肿瘤术后神经功能的评估缺乏一个广泛认同的标准，大多数研究仅仅使用正常或异常来描述患者的功能状态，无法准确反映患者术后的神经功能结局。1997 年，Biagini 等提出了一个评分系统，这个评分系统包括排尿功能、排便功能和下肢活动 3 项内容，每项内容根据患者情况分为 0 分、1 分、2 分。该评分系统对这个领域的发展做出积极的贡献，后来 Fourney 等和 Moran 等发表的一系列的研究都采用了这个评分系统。但这个评分系统还不足以对骶骨切除术后患者的神经功能进行定量分析。2016 年黄林等在 Biagini 的评分系统的基础上进行了拓展，提出了一个新的评分系统。这个系统包括排尿功能、排便功能和下肢功能 3 个领域，每个领域再细分出 3 个项目，根据患者情况每个项目分为 0 分、1 分、2 分、3 分。相比之下，黄林等提出的评分系统内容更加充分翔实，区分度更高，能定量描述骶骨肿瘤术后患者的神经功能状态。

全骶骨切除术是治疗骶骨高位原发性恶性骨肿瘤的主要手段，目前已有不少文献对不同切除水平的骶骨切除术后患者的神经功能进行研究，但由于病例的缺乏，针对全骶骨切除术后患者的神经功能结局的研究还很少。全骶骨切除术后的神经功能结局对于评价患者整体预后具有非常重要的意义，对于决定手术方案时的术后功能预测具有重要的参考价值。因此，全骶骨切除术后患者的神经功能水平还有待相关学者进行更多的探讨。

1.3 全骶骨切除术后患者的健康相关生命质量

20 世纪 50 年代以来，慢性非传染性疾病逐渐替代传染性疾病成为人类死亡的主要原因，指导现代医学理论与实践的范式也从生物医学理论逐渐转变为生物—心理—社会医学模式。世界卫生组织提出："健康不仅仅是没有疾病或虚弱的状态，而是生理、心理和社会方面的完好状态。"因此，仅以复发率、死亡率和病死率作为疾病的预后指标具有很大的局限性。自 20 世纪 70 年代末起，医学领域开始引入生命质量概念，将生命质量当作评价医疗水平的重要指标，形成了相关生命质量研究领域。

健康相关生命质量是一种新的健康评价技术，它在特定的文化和价值体系中，在疾病及医疗干预的影响下，测定与患者个人生活事件相联系的主观健康状态和个体满意度。健康相关生命质量对患者进行了充分的评价，包括疾病及治疗对患者造成的生理、心理和社会生活等方面的影响。它既关心患者的存活时间，又关心患者的存活质量；既考虑客观的指标，又强调患者的主观感受。传统医疗保健评价方法往往局限于生命的存活时间和局部功能的改善，无法全面评估健康结局，而健康相关生命质量则有效弥补了这个缺点。

健康相关生命质量是重要的卫生保健信息，它在评定人群健康状况、评估疾病负担、比较临床治疗方法、选择患者治疗方案以及决策卫生资源的配置和利用等方面都有广泛的应用。健康相关生命质量评价符合以患者为中心的健康服务趋势，它能帮助医生探索最优化的治疗结局，帮助研究者评价新的治疗方案和技术，帮助管理者追求卫生投入效用最大化，帮助患者比较不同医疗卫生服务的成本和效益，以弥补卫生保健信息不对称造成的卫生服务需方和卫生服务供方之间的裂痕。

由于切除了 S1 及以下神经，全骶骨切除术会对患者的下肢功能、大小便功能和性功能造成严重损害，这不仅严重影响患者的生理功能，也对患者的心理和社会生活造成了严重的困扰。因此，评价全骶骨切除术后患者的健康相关生命质量，对全面评估这类患者的整体预后而言是不可或缺的重要组成部分，有利于充分评估者进行全骶骨切除术的成本与获益，对于医疗决策具有重要的参考价值。

然而，有关全骶骨切除术后患者健康相关生命质量的文献是极其罕见的。2016 年，Phukan 等使用患者报告结局测量信息系统（Patient-reported Outcome Measurement Information System，PROMIS）对 33 例不同切除水平的骶骨切除术后患者进行了健康相关生命质量的评估，平均随访时间 41 个月，发现骶骨切除术的截骨水平越高，术后患者的健康相关生命质量越低，其中的 6 例全骶骨切除术后患者在所有研究对象中的健康相关生命质量是最低的。除此以外，并没有发现其他文献对全骶骨切除术后患者的健康相关生命质量进行研究。

对全骶骨切除术后患者的健康相关生命质量进行研究，需要选择一个合适的生命质量量表。由于该领域的相关文献太少，因此笔者参考了关于脊柱肿瘤患者术后的健康相关生命质量的相关文献，发现有关学者使用的工具有 SF-36（the medical outcomes study 36-item short form health survey，SF-36）量表、PROMIS 系统、欧洲五维健康量表（EuroQol Five Dimensions Questionnaire，EQ-5D）、Owestry 功能障碍指数（Owestry disability index，ODI）、KPS 评分（Karnofsky Performance Status，KPS）、美国东部肿瘤合作组织评分（Eastern Cooperative Oncology Group，ECOG）量表等。这些量表都是国外的学者进行研究制作的，由于不同国家之间的文化差异以及不同国家人群的健康水平之间的差异，如果在我国使用这些量表进行研究，为了保证研究结果的严谨和准确，一般需要对量表进行翻译，并针对我国人群的特点进行性能测试和常模制订。其中，2003 年浙江大学李鲁教授等对 SF-36 量表针对中国人群进行了性能测试和常模制订，因此，SF-36 量表便直接应用于中国患者的临床研究。和其他生命质量量表相比，SF-36 量表短小、灵活、易管理，信度和效度令人满意，具有较高的敏感性。作为一个简单明了的健康调查问卷，它一共有 36 个问题，从生理功能、生理职能、躯体疼痛、总体健康状况、活力、社会功能、情感职能以及精神健康等 8 个方面全面概括了被调查者的生存质量，有利于全面评估全骶骨切除术后患者的健康相关生命质量。

总而言之，研究全骶骨切除术后患者的健康相关生命质量具有非常重要的价值，而该领域的相关文献还相当罕见，国内还没有学者进行这方面的研究，仍待有关学者进行更多相关的研究，以填补这方面的空白。

1.4　全骶骨切除术后患者的生活和情感体验

上文提到，全骶骨切除术后患者的下肢功能、大小便功能和性功能都会受到严重的损伤，该手术属于致残性手术。因此，骶骨肿瘤以及手术的治疗会对患者及其家人的生活造成很大的影响，他们基本上很难回归到患病前的生活状态，这类患者与其他部位肿瘤的患者相比有相对独特的术后生活经历和情感体验。

通过查阅现有的文献发现，几乎没有文献报道这类患者术后的生活经历和情感体验。2010 年，Davidge 等采用定性分析的方法对 12 例骶骨肿瘤术后患者进行研究，他们对每一个患者单独进行半结构化访谈，平均访谈时间为 34 分钟，访谈的内容主要为以下 5 个主题：①手术对患者及其家人生活的影响；②患者对住院期间治疗的满意程度；③与骶骨相关的慢性疼痛；④患者对远期康复信息的需求；⑤患者对活着的感激态度。这个研究发现，骶骨肿瘤术后的患者及其家人的生活都发生了很大的改变，并且他们需要更多远期康复治疗的信息。可惜的是，这个研究中的 12 例患者都是 S1 以下神经水平截骨的患者，并没有全骶骨切除术的病例。2016 年，Barsan 等对一个骶骨肌纤维母细胞肉瘤行全骶骨切除术的年轻女性做了一个个案分析，随访时间为 5 年，患者没有肿瘤复发和疼痛的困扰，依靠踝关节矫正器能独立行走，最可喜的是患者术后顺利走进婚姻的殿堂并且正常怀孕，在孕 37 周的时候通过选择性剖宫产的方式顺利分娩出一个女婴，孩子生长非常健康。除此以外，没有其他文献对全骶骨切除术后患者的生活体验进行报道。

定性分析的方法能够深入探讨患者的个人体验，有利于评估疾病对患者个人生活和情感体验的影响。有文献报道对骨盆肿瘤和肢体骨肉瘤的患者用定性分析的方法进行患者术后生活经历和情感体验的研究，取得了良好的研究效果。

研究患者术后的生活经历和情感体验，能够让医生和其他医疗工作人员更好地理解患者在全骶骨切除术后的生理、心理、社会和情感经历，将使外科医生和其他保健工作者更好地指导手术决策，管理患者围手术期的期望，并更好地协助患者康复。国内外的学者还没有针对全骶骨切除术后患者在术后生活经历和情感体验进行系统的研究，所以需要引起有关学者对这方面的兴趣，并加以研究，从而填补这个领域的空白。

2　研究目的与意义

2.1　研究目的

2.1.1　研究全骶骨切除术后患者的外科治疗结局

统计全骶骨切除术后患者的肿瘤学预后、围手术期并发症，评估患者的神经功能结局。

2.1.2　研究全骶骨切除术后患者的健康相关生命质量

使用 SF-36 量表对患者进行健康相关生命质量评估，引入社会经济地位评分、神经功能评分、肿瘤学预后、围手术期并发症等因素，探索全骶骨切除术后患者健康相关生命质量的影响因素。

2.1.3　研究全骶骨切除术后患者的生活及情感体验

采用半结构化访谈的方式深入探讨全骶骨切除术后患者的个人体验，定性分析全骶骨切除术后患者的生活经历和情感体验。

2.2　研究背景及意义

全骶骨切除术是高位骶骨恶性肿瘤的主要治疗方法。全骶骨切除术由于完全切除患者 S1 及以下神经，会对患者的下肢功能、大小便功能和性功能造成永久的损害，属于致残性手术，对患者的生理、心理、社会功能和情感体验都会产生显著的影响。

既往文献报道了全骶骨切除术后患者的手术并发症、神经功能损伤及肿瘤学预后。但既往文献报道的病例数都比较少，需要更多病例的数据以获得更准确的结论。另外，罕有文献报道全骶骨切除术后患者的健康相关生命质量，还没有学者对全骶骨切除术后患者的生活经历和情感体验进行定性分析。因此，本研究可以填补骨肿瘤学科在这个方面的空白，对骨肿瘤学科的发展具有非常重要的研究价值。

研究全骶骨切除术后患者的外科治疗结局、健康相关生命质量以及患者的生活经历和情感体验，有利于全面评价全骶骨切除术的成本与获益，能使外科医生和其他保健工作者更好地指导手术决策，管理患者围手术期的期望，并更好地协助患者康复。

2.3 研究方法

2.3.1 调查对象

患者的纳入标准：曾于本中心行全骶骨切除术，可查到完整的电子病历，能通过电话联系上并且愿意参与本次研究的患者。

排除标准：已经死亡的患者；失访患者；不愿意参与本次研究的患者。

2.3.2 调查方法

通过查阅本中心既往电子病历，找出曾于我中心行全骶骨切除术的患者资料，通过电话号码联系患者，将能够联系上并愿意参与本次调查的患者进行登记入组。

通过查阅既往电子病历，统计患者的首发症状、病例类型、住院时间、是否初次手术、手术出血量、手术并发症等信息。

制作调查问卷，内容主要包括年龄、性别、文化程度、职业、家庭人均收入以及中文版 SF-36 v2 量表。使用问卷星软件制作网上调查问卷，通过电子邮件或微信发给患者，让患者在网上进行填写和提交。对于部分不懂得使用电脑或智能手机的患者，让其家属协助其填写问卷。

与患者约定好时间，通过电话访谈的方式，对患者进行半结构化访谈，访谈的主题内容包括：①日常生活能力；②社会交际情况；③学习或工作情况；④对家庭的影响；⑤对造瘘手术的接受程度；⑥对远期康复指导的需求；⑦对住院期间医疗服务的满意度；⑧对治疗结局的满意度。

2.3.3 数据处理

使用 SPSS 20.0 进行数据分析。

3 全骶骨切除术后患者的外科治疗结局及健康相关生命质量

3.1 前言

骶骨肿瘤比较少见，约占原发性骨肿瘤的 1% ～ 3.5%，其中以脊索瘤最多见，其次为骨巨细胞瘤。原发高度恶性骨肿瘤更为少见，主要包括骨肉瘤、软骨肉瘤、尤因肉瘤等。对于骶骨的原发性恶性骨肿瘤，为了保证足够的外科边界，降低局部复发率，达到治愈的目的，必须行广泛性切除手术。目前，对于累及 S2 及以上神经的高位骶骨恶性肿瘤，临床上主要的治疗手段是全骶骨切除术。

既往文献报道了全骶骨切除术后患者的手术并发症、神经功能损伤及肿瘤学预后。然而，大多数研究往往侧重于患者的肿瘤学预后，对患者的功能结局也只是简单的描述，几乎没有文献对骶骨肿瘤术后患者的健康相关生命质量进行报道，所以无法全面评估患者的预后。全骶骨切除术作为致残性手术，会严重影响患者的生理、心理和社会功能。因此，评价全骶骨切除术后患者的健康相关生命质量，有利于充分评估患者进行全骶骨切除术的成本与获益，有利于对患者做出一个全面、彻底且便于理解的解释，对于医生和患者进行医疗决策具有重要的参考价值。

本研究的目的是回顾全骶骨切除术后患者的肿瘤学预后、手术并发症，以及评估患者的神经功能结局和健康相关生命质量，并分析健康相关生命质量的影响因素。

3.2　研究对象及研究方法

3.2.1　研究对象

通过查阅本中心既往电子病历，找出 2007 年 9 月—2017 年 9 月曾于本中心行全骶骨切除术的患者的资料，发现共有 52 例患者曾于本中心行全骶骨肿瘤切除术，通过电子病历上留下的联系方式，对患者或其家属进行电话联系，有 11 例患者失访，有 8 例患者已经死亡（均死于肿瘤的复发与转移），剩下的 33 例患者均可正常随访并愿意参与本次研究。在这 33 例患者中，共有男性 18 例、女性 15 例，平均年龄 47.4 岁（范围 13～75 岁），具体分布见图 3.1。

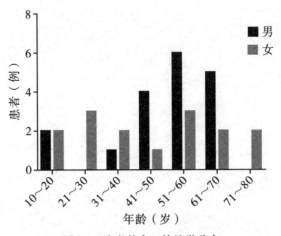

图 3.1　患者的人口统计学分布

患者的病理类型，主要以脊索瘤（21 例）为主，其次为软骨肉瘤（5 例）、骨肉瘤（3 例）、尤因肉瘤（2 例）、神经鞘瘤（1 例）、结肠癌（1 例），其百分比构成见图 3.2。在这些患者中，有 11 例患者为术后复发再次手术，剩余的 22 例患者为初次手术。患者发病时的首发症状，主要表现为骶尾部疼痛（25例），其次为大便障碍（3例）、下肢麻木（2例）、下肢疼痛（1例）、臀部麻木（1例）、小便障碍（1例）。

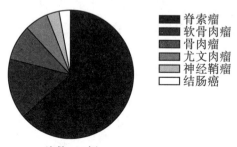

脊索瘤
软骨肉瘤
骨肉瘤
尤文肉瘤
神经鞘瘤
结肠癌

总数=33例

图 3.2　患者的病理类型构成

3.2.2　研究方法

患者于本中心就诊时，除了进行病史采集和体格检查，还进行术前评估，一般包括平片、CT、MRI、骨扫描，部分患者会在术前进行穿刺活检。手术时常规对患者行腹主动脉球囊阻断，以减少患者术中出血。手术入路采取单纯后侧（24例）或前后侧联合入路（9例），术中从L5/S1椎间盘离断，将整块骶骨切除，然后使用钉棒系统重建骶髂关节（图3.3）。

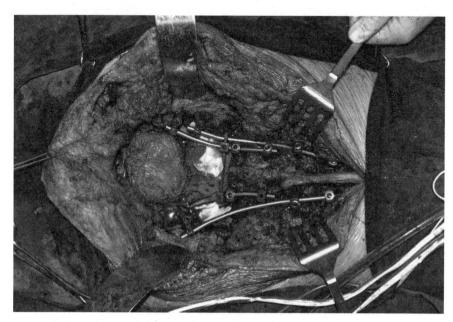

图 3.3　全骶骨切除术关伤口前

骨肉瘤患者和尤因肉瘤患者常规行术前化疗和术后化疗，其他病理类型的患者均未行化疗。所有患者平均住院时间（不包括化疗时间）为 37 天（范围 18 ～ 75 天），住院时间的分布见图 3.4。

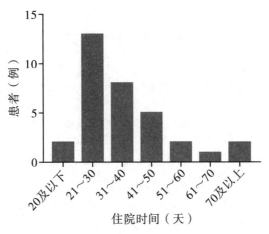

图 3.4　患者住院时间的分布情况

所有患者平均随访时间为 25 个月（范围 4 ～ 93 个月），将不同随访时间的患者进行分组，其分布见图 3.5。

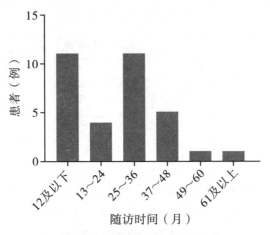

图 3.5　患者的随访时间分布

本次随访过程从 2017 年 11 月 1 日开始至 2018 年 1 月 31 日结束，为期 3 个月。通过查阅既往电子病历，统计患者的首发症状、病理类型、住院时间、是否初次手术、手术出血量、手术并发症（包括伤口并发症、脑脊液漏、肠道损伤、内固定失败）等信息。

通过电话随访，仔细询问患者下肢功能和大小便功能，包括下肢疼痛、下肢运动、会阴感觉、排尿困难、尿失禁、膀胱感觉、便秘、大便失禁、直肠感觉等情况，并使用黄林等建立的骶骨切除术后神经功能评分系统对患者进行评分，具体见表3.1。

表3.1　骶骨切除术后神经功能评分系统

项目	表现	3分	2分	1分	0分
下肢运动和感觉	运动	正常	轻度损伤，行走不需要外部支持	行走需要外部支持（如手杖、拐杖等）	移动需要轮椅/卧床
	疼痛	无	轻度疼痛，不需要使用镇痛药	中度疼痛，可通过镇痛药控制	难治性疼痛/药物依赖
	会阴感觉	正常	轻度麻木或感觉过敏，不影响日常生活	麻木或感觉过敏，影响日常生活	会阴感觉完全丧失
排尿功能和膀胱感觉	排尿困难	正常	轻度排尿困难，不需要用手挤压腹部或医疗干预	需要用手挤压腹部或偶尔导尿（每周少于1次）	尿潴留，需要留置尿管或常规间歇导尿/完全尿失禁/输尿管造瘘
	尿失禁	正常	偶尔漏尿，不需要使用尿布	频繁漏尿，需要常规使用尿布	留置尿管/完全尿失禁/输尿管造瘘
	膀胱感觉	正常	轻度改变，但排尿时仍存在膀胱感觉	有时会丧失对排尿的感觉刺激	完全丧失对排尿的感觉刺激/留置尿管/输尿管造瘘
排便功能和直肠感觉	便秘	正常	轻度排便困难，不需要医疗干预	中度排便困难，需要经常使用灌肠剂或导泄	排便困难，需要用手协助排便/完全便秘/结肠造瘘
	大便失禁	正常	偶尔失禁，不需要使用尿布	频繁失禁，需要常规使用尿布	完全失禁/结肠造瘘
	直肠感觉	正常	减弱但排便时仍存在	有时丧失对排便的感觉刺激	完全丧失对排便的感觉刺激/结肠造瘘

使用中文版SF-36 v2量表对患者进行健康相关生命质量的评估。SF-36量表是1988年美国波士顿健康研究所在医疗机构研究调查表（medical outcomes study，MOS）的基础上开发的通用性简明健康调查问卷。后来Ware等对SF-36量表进行了修改，建立了SF-36 v2量表，调整了问卷布局，简化了条目用词，修改了部分条目的选项数，并实行了基于常模的记分规则。2009年，某学者针对中国人群对SF-36 v2量表进行了性能测试和常模制订。SF-36 v2量表共有36个条目，通过8个维度评价健康相关生命质量：生理功能（physical function，PF）、生理职能（role-physical，RP）、躯体疼痛（bodily pain，BP）、总体健康（general

health，GH）、活力（vitality，VT）、社会功能（social function，SF）、情感职能
（role-emotional，RE）和精神健康（mental health，MH）。在 8 个维度的得分基础
上，可分别计算生理健康总分（physical component summary，PCS）和心理健康总
分（mental component summary，MCS）。

制作调查问卷，内容主要包括年龄、性别、文化程度、职业、家庭人均收入
以及中文版 SF-36 v2 量表（见附录 1）。使用问卷星软件制作网上调查问卷，通
过电子邮件或微信发给患者，让患者在网上进行填写和提交。对于部分不懂得使
用电脑或智能手机的患者，让其家属协助其填写问卷。

回收问卷后，按照 SF-36 v2 量表的记分规则，计算各维度的原始分数，然
后折算成转换分数。将条目选项转换成条目分数时，条目 1、6、7、8、9a、9d、
9e、9h、11b、11d 为逆向条目，分数应作正向变换；其余条目为正向条目，分
数保持不变。如表 3.2 所示，先对同一维度的全部条目分数进行求和，计算维度
原始分数。最后再用极差法计算各维度的转换分：转换分 = ［（原始分数 – 最低
可能分数）÷（最高可能分数 – 最低可能分数）］× 100。通过各个分项目的分数
可以计算生理健康总分（PCS）和心理健康总分（MCS）：

$$PCS = PH \times（0.430）+ RP \times（0.344）+ BP \times（0.300）+ GH \times（0.205）$$
$$+ VT \times（0.019）+ SF \times（0.087）+ RE \times（-0.177）+ MH \times（-0.285）;$$

$$MCS = PH \times（-0.262）+ RP \times（-0.145）+ BP \times（-0.111）+ GH \times（0.018）$$
$$+ VT \times（0.234）+ SF \times（0.153）+ RE \times（0.437）+ MH \times（0.559）。$$

表 3.2　SF-36 v2 量表各维度原始分数计分方法

维度	条目数	计分方法	得分范围（分）
生理功能（PF）	10	3a+3b+3c+3d+3e+3f+3g+3h+3i+3g	10～30
生理职能（RP）	4	4a+4b+4c+4d	4～20
躯体疼痛（BP）	2	7+8	2～11
总体健康（GH）	5	1+11a+11b+11c+11d	5～25
活力（VT）	4	9a+9e+9g+9i	4～20
社会功能（SF）	2	6+10	2～10
情感职能（RE）	3	5a+5b+5c	3～15
精神健康（MH）	5	9b+9c+9d+9f+9h	5～25

引入中国社会经济地位指数，分析全骶骨切除术后患者健康相关生命质量的
影响因素。采用清华大学教授李强建立的中国大城市居民经济地位量表，通过文
化程度、职业和家庭人均收入 3 个方面对患者的社会经济地位进行评估。在该表

中（见表3.3），教育程度从不识字或识字很少到硕士研究生毕业及以上，分别评分为1～7分；考虑到个人收入受到家庭其他成员收入和消费的影响，所以该量表使用的是家庭成员人均月收入指标，以人民币"元"为单位，从500元及500元以下到6001元及6001元以上分别评分为1～7分；职业从临时工、进城务工人员、无职业者到高层管理人员与高级专业技术人员分别评分为1～7分。教育、家庭人均月收入和职业三者得分相加获得总分，总分最低为3分，最高为21分。

表3.3　中国大城市居民社会经济地位量表

教育、收入与职业	项目	得分（分）
教育	硕士研究生毕业及以上	7
	大学本科毕业	6
	大学专科毕业	5
	高中、中专、中技、职高毕业	4
	初中毕业	3
	小学毕业	2
	不识字或识字很少	1
家庭人均月收入	≥6001元	7
	4001～6000元	6
	3001～4000元	5
	2001～3000元	4
	1001～2000元	3
	501～1000元	2
	≤500元	1
职业	高层管理人员与高级专业技术人员	7
	中层管理人员与中级专业技术人员	6
	一般管理人员与一般专业技术人员	5
	办公室一般工作人员	4
	技术工人	3
	体力劳动工人	2
	临时工、进城务工人员、无职业者	1

对参与本研究的33例患者的社会经济地位评分进行计算并分组，其结果如图3.6所示。

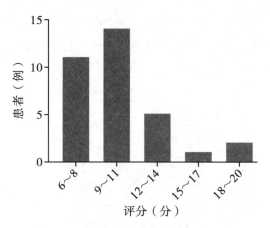

图 3.6　患者社会经济地位评分的分布

3.3　研究结果

3.3.1　手术并发症

患者术中出血平均值为 2771 mL（范围 800 ～ 9000 mL），将不同出血量的患者进行分组，患者的出血量集中分布在 1000 ～ 4000 mL 之间，具体分布见图 3.7。

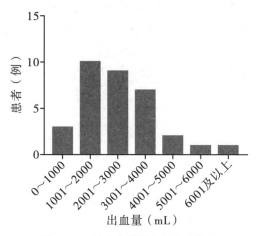

图 3.7　不同出血量的患者分布情况

在这 33 例患者中，出现术后并发症包括伤口并发症、内固定失败、脑脊液漏、肠道损伤这 4 种，详见图 3.8。伤口并发症的患者共 14 例，这些患者均进行了清创手术，清创术后患者伤口基本愈合良好，但有 1 例患者经过 2 次清创手术后伤口仍未愈合，患者出院后一直定期换药，至参加此次随访时伤口仍未愈合。内固定失败患者 7 例，其中 5 例进行了内固定翻修手术，1 例进行了内固定取出旷置处理，1 例未予处理。脑脊液漏患者 6 例，其中 5 例患者经过使用抗生素、抬高床尾等治疗后好转，1 例患者保守治疗无效，行修补手术后好转。出现肠道损伤均行结肠造瘘手术的患者 2 例。

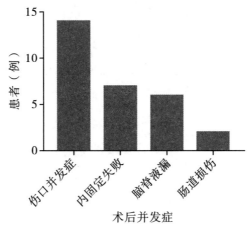

图 3.8　患者术后并发症的情况

3.3.2　肿瘤学预后

2009 年 9 月—2017 年 9 月期间曾在本中心行全骶骨切除术的 52 例患者中，除了失访的 11 例患者，剩下的 41 例患者中，共有 13 例患者复发，平均复发时间为 11.5 个月（范围 3 ～ 24 个月），其中患者已经死亡 8 例，平均死亡时间为 42 个月（范围 10 ～ 96 个月）。将这 41 例患者的复发和死亡情况做成复发曲线和生存曲线，分别见图 3.9 和图 3.10。

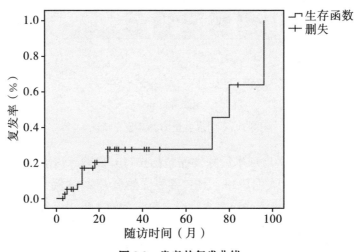

图 3.9　患者的复发曲线

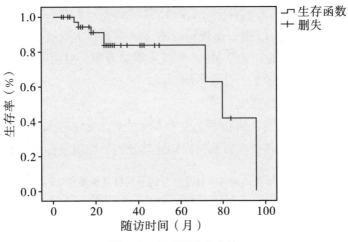

图 3.10　患者的生存曲线

3.3.3　神经功能结局

使用黄林等建立的骶骨切除术后神经功能评估系统，从下肢运动、下肢疼痛、会阴感觉、排尿困难、尿失禁、膀胱感觉、便秘、大便失禁、直肠感觉等9 个方面，对患者的神经功能结局进行评估。

（1）下肢运动和感觉

下肢运动和感觉包括运动、疼痛、会阴感觉 3 个项目，各个项目以及下肢功能总分的平均值及标准差见表 3.4。

表3.4　下肢功能各项目及总分的平均值及标准差（$\bar{x} \pm s$，分）

组别	运动	疼痛	会阴感觉	下肢功能总分
无复发证据组	1.57±0.88	1.21±0.57	1.08±0.69	3.86±1.65
复发组	0.40±0.90	0.40±0.90	0.40±0.90	1.20±2.17

28 例无复发证据组的患者中，出现无法行走的情况 2 例，他们长期卧床，移动时需要家属协助使用轮椅；行走时需要助步器、拐杖等外部支持 18 例；行走功能轻度损伤，但不需要使用拐杖等外部支持 8 例；没有下肢运动功能完全恢复正常的患者。5 例复发组的患者中，长期卧床 4 例，行走时需使用助步器 1 例。

28 例无复发证据组的患者中，出现了难治性的疼痛或因疼痛引起了药物依赖 2 例；出现了中度疼痛，通过镇痛药控制效果良好 13 例；出现了轻度疼痛，不需要使用镇痛药即可忍受 8 例；无疼痛症状 5 例。5 例复发组患者中，出现了难治性的疼痛或因疼痛引起了药物依赖 4 例，出现了不需使用镇痛药的轻度疼痛1 例。

28 例无复发证据组的患者中，会阴感觉完全丧失 8 例；出现会阴感觉麻木或过敏，影响日常生活 12 例；出现轻度的会阴感觉麻木或过敏，但不影响日常生活 6 例；自述会阴感觉正常 2 例。5 例复发组患者中，会阴感觉完全消失 4 例，出现会阴感觉麻木或过敏影响日常生活 1 例。

（2）排尿功能和膀胱感觉

从排尿困难、尿失禁、膀胱感觉 3 个方面对全骶骨切除术后患者的排尿功能和排尿感觉进行评估，各个项目及排尿功能总分的平均值及标准差见表 3.5。

表3.5　患者排尿功能各项目及总分的平均值及标准差（$\bar{x} \pm s$，分）

组别	排尿困难	尿失禁	膀胱感觉	排尿功能总分
无复发证据组	1.43±0.88	1.29±0.71	1.07±0.90	3.79±2.08
复发组	0.20±0.45	0.20±0.45	0.20±0.45	0.60±1.34

在排尿困难方面，28 例无复发证据组的患者中，需要长期留置尿管或已行输尿管造瘘 4 例，因排尿困难需常规间歇导尿 1 例；出现较严重的排尿困难，排尿时需要用手挤压腹部，以增加腹压辅助排尿 8 例；出现轻度的排尿困难，平时排尿不需要用手挤压腹部或采用其他医疗干预手段 13 例；自述排尿完全正常 2 例。在 5 例复发组的患者中，需要长期留置尿管或已行输尿管造瘘 4 例；出现较严重的排尿困难，排尿时需要用手挤压腹部 1 例。

在尿失禁方面，28 例无复发证据组的患者中，需要长期留置尿管或已行输尿管造瘘 4 例；漏尿情况频繁，日常生活中需要经常使用尿布 12 例；偶尔会出现漏尿，但日常生活中不需要使用尿布 12 例；没有患者自述未出现漏尿情况。在 5 例复发组的患者中，需要长期留置尿管或已行输尿管造瘘 4 例；偶尔出现漏尿，平时不需要使用尿布 1 例。

在膀胱感觉方面，28 例无复发证据组的患者中，完全丧失对排尿的感觉刺激 5 例，需要长期留置尿管或行输尿管造瘘 4 例；排尿时有时可以感觉排尿的感觉，但有时又会丧失排尿的感觉 9 例；排尿时的膀胱感觉出现轻度异常，但在排尿时均存在膀胱感觉 9 例；自述排尿时膀胱感觉完全正常 1 例。在 5 例复发组的患者中，需要长期留置尿管或行输尿管造瘘 4 例；有时会丧失排尿的感觉 1 例。

（3）排便功能和直肠感觉

从便秘、大便失禁、直肠感觉 3 个方面对全骶骨切除术后患者的排便功能和直肠感觉进行评估，各个项目及排便功能总分的平均值及标准差见表 3.6。

表3.6 排便功能各项目及总分的平均值及标准差（$\bar{x} \pm s$，分）

组别	便秘	大便失禁	直肠感觉异常	排便功能总分
无复发证据组	1.29±0.76	1.68±0.72	1.04±0.74	4.01±1.93
复发组	0.20±0.45	0.20±0.45	0.40±0.90	0.80±0.84

在便秘方面，28 例无复发证据组的患者中，出现严重的排便困难，需要用手协助排便或已行结肠造瘘 4 例；出现中度排便困难，需要经常使用灌肠剂，或使用药物进行导泄 13 例；出现轻度的排便困难，但不需要灌肠或者导泄等医疗干预手段 10 例；自述排便时完全正常，未出现排便困难 1 例。在 5 例复发组的患者中，出现严重的排便困难，需要用手协助排便或已行结肠造瘘 4 例；出现轻度的排便困难，但不需要灌肠或者导泄等医疗干预手段 1 例。

在大便失禁方面，28 例无复发证据组的患者中，出现完全大便失禁或已行结肠造瘘 2 例；频繁出现大便失禁的情况，日常生活中需要常规使用垫布 7 例；偶尔会出现大便失禁的情况，但平时不需要常规使用垫布 17 例；自述未出现大便失禁情况 2 例。在 5 例复发组的患者中，出现完全大便失禁或已行结肠造瘘 4 例；偶尔会出现大便失禁的情况，但平时不需要常规使用垫布 1 例。

在直肠感觉方面，28 例无复发证据组的患者中，完全丧失了对排便的感觉刺激或已行结肠造瘘 7 例；部分时间在排便时可以感觉到大便对直肠的刺激，部分时间则完全丧失对排便的感觉 13 例；直肠感觉出现轻度改变，但排便时均能感觉到大便对直肠的刺激 8 例；没有患者自述直肠感觉完全恢复正常。在 5 例复发组的患者中，完全丧失直肠感觉或已行结肠造瘘 4 例；出现轻度的直肠感觉改变 1 例。

（4）神经功能总体情况

分析 28 例无复发证据组患者在下肢运动、下肢疼痛、会阴感觉、排尿困难、尿失禁、膀胱感觉、便秘、大便失禁、直肠感觉等 9 个项目不同得分所占百分比的情况，详见图 3.10。

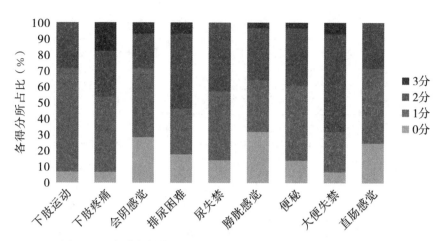

图 3.8　无复发证据组患者神经功能评分各个项目得分占比情况

将 9 个项目的得分进行求和，即可得到无复发证据组患者和复发组患者神经功能评分的总分（见表 3.7）。

表 3.7　无复发证据组和复发组患者神经功能评分得分情况（$\bar{x} \pm s$，分）

组别	下肢功能总分	排尿功能总分	排便功能总分	神经功能总分
无复发证据组	3.86±1.65	3.79±2.08	4.01±1.93	11.66±4.65
复发组	1.20±2.17	0.60±1.34	0.80±0.84	2.60±2.88

3.3.4　健康相关生命质量

通过 SF-36 v2 量表评分，得到了全骶骨切除术后患者生理功能、生理职能、躯体疼痛、总体健康、活力、社会功能、情感职能和精神健康 8 个维度的得分，并在此基础上计算出了生理健康总分和心理健康总分。表 3.8 则描述了无复发证据组、复发组的各个维度以及生理健康总分和心理健康总分的平均分及标准差，并引入了中国普通人群常模得分进行对比。

从表 3.8 可以看到，无论是 SF-36 v2 量表的 8 个维度还是生理健康总分和心理健康总分，无复发证据组和复发组的得分与中国普通人群常模相比都有显著的下降，而且复发组患者的得分要远远低于无复发证据组患者的。对比生理健康总分和心理健康总分的情况，可以看到无复发证据组和复发组患者在生理健康总分方面的下降要比心理健康总分方面的下降更加明显，说明骶骨肿瘤以及全骶骨切除术的治疗，对患者在生理健康方面的影响大于心理健康方面的影响。

表 3.8　无复发证据组和复发组患者及中国普通人群各项目的平均分及标准差（$\bar{x} \pm s$，分）

项目	无复发证据组	复发组	中国普通人群常模
生理功能	38.93 ± 28.16	7.50 ± 11.18	87.6 ± 16.8
生理职能	30.05 ± 27.33	0.00 ± 0.00	83.0 ± 20.7
躯体疼痛	43.30 ± 20.62	4.44 ± 2.79	83.3 ± 19.7
总体健康	39.46 ± 21.96	15.00 ± 17.32	68.2 ± 19.4
活力	43.31 ± 20.62	30.00 ± 24.37	70.1 ± 16.8
社会功能	38.04 ± 27.72	7.50 ± 11.78	84.8 ± 16.6
情感职能	47.91 ± 24.50	6.67 ± 14.90	85.3 ± 17.7
精神健康	57.14 ± 19.12	41.00 ± 26.79	78.8 ± 15.4
生理健康总分	30.37 ± 25.58	−6.37 ± 3.15	76.34 ± 18.72
心理健康总分	49.13 ± 18.98	33.25 ± 23.36	67.7 ± 16.81

3.3.5　健康相关生命质量的影响因素

为研究全骶骨切除术后患者健康相关生命质量的影响因素，使用统计学方法对年龄、性别、社会经济地位评分、病理类型、出血量、手术并发症、手术入路、神经功能评分等因素进行了分析。为了排除肿瘤复发因素的影响，这里的分析只涉及无复发证据组的患者。

针对性别、有无伤口并发症、有无内固定失败、有无脑脊液漏、手术入路是单纯后路还是前后路联合，对患者分别进行两两分组，然后使用曼–惠特尼（Mann-Whitney）U 检验比较两组数据之间的差异。表 3.9 对性别、手术并发症、手术入路进行分组后，分别针对生理健康总分和心理健康总分进行 Mann-Whitney U 检验，结果显示，所有 P 值均大于 0.05，说明性别、伤口并发症、内固定失败、脑脊液漏以及手术入路因素对全骶骨切除术后患者的生理健康总分和心理健康总分的影响均没有统计学差异。

表 3.9　Mann-Whitney U 检验的结果

项目	生理健康总分	心理健康总分
性别	0.205	0.420
伤口并发症	0.767	0.521
内固定失败	0.453	0.741
脑脊液漏	0.480	0.472
手术入路	0.326	0.160

通过 Kruskal-Wallis 检验方法分析不同病理类型对生理健康总分和心理健康总分的影响，得到的结果如表 3.10 所示。结果显示，P 值均大于 0.05，说明病理类型对生理健康总分和心理健康总分的影响没有统计学差异。

表 3.10　Kruskal-Wallis 检验的结果

	生理健康总分	心理健康总分
P 值	0.440	0.454

通过 Spearman 相关性分析研究年龄、社会经济地位评分、出血量和神经功能评分总分对生理健康总分和心理健康总分的影响，得到的结果如表 3.11 所示。

由表 3.11 可以得知，年龄、社会经济地位评分以及出血量均与生理健康总分或心理健康总分之间没有显著相关。

表 3.11　Spearman 相关性的结果

项目	生理健康总分		心理健康总分	
	r 值	P 值	r 值	P 值
年龄	−0.375	0.490	0.017	0.932
社会经济地位评分	0.406	0.320	0.133	0.499
出血量	0.110	0.578	0.019	0.924
神经功能评分总分	0.867	<0.001	0.520	0.005

图 3.10 和图 3.11 分别描述了神经功能评分总分与生理健康总分及心理健康总分之间的相关性。神经功能评分总分与生理健康总分存在相关性，呈高度正相关；神经功能评分总分与心理健康总分存在相关性，呈中度正相关。

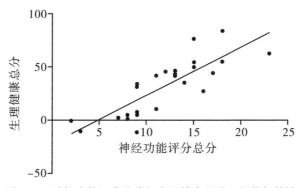

图 3.10　神经功能评分总分与生理健康总分之间的相关性

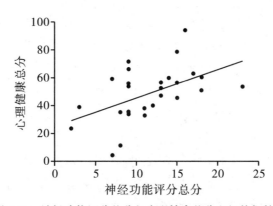

图 3.11　神经功能评分总分与生理健康总分之间的相关性

3.4　讨论

3.4.1　手术并发症的原因与防治

参与本次研究的全骶骨切除术后患者，曾经出现过的手术并发症包括术中大量出血、伤口并发症、内固定失败、脑脊液漏、肠道损伤等，与以往文献报道的相似。

骶骨肿瘤往往肿瘤体积巨大，局部解剖结构复杂，局部血液供应丰富，且术中止血困难，因此术中出血往往较多。高位骶骨肿瘤位置离头端更近，相比其他水平的骶骨切除手术，高位骶骨肿瘤的切除手术需要暴露的部位更多，因此行全骶骨切除手术时出血量往往也更大。术中大量出血不仅容易引起失血性休克，增加围手术期并发症的发生率及死亡率，而且容易造成术野不清，肿瘤切除不彻底，增加肿瘤的复发率。为了减少手术出血，1975 年 Feldman 等提出可以在术前行双侧髂内动脉及肿瘤供血血管的栓塞，作为控制术中出血的手段，但相关文献报道单纯行血管栓塞术控制出血效果不满意。如果在术中行腹主动脉临时阻断，控制出血效果较好，但必须先行前路手术，由此增加了手术时间和手术创伤，且患者体位须为侧卧位，在后路切除肿瘤时影响视野的暴露。文献报道使用腹主动脉球囊阻断技术控制骶骨手术出血有令人满意的效果。腹主动脉球囊阻断技术，即在术前应用血管造影技术，在腹主动脉预先留置球囊，如果在术中出现较大的手术出血，则通过向球囊内注入生理盐水充盈球囊，起到临时阻断腹主动脉的作用。本研究中的 33 例患者均采用了腹主动脉球囊阻断技术控制手术出血，平均出血量为 2771 mL，与 Fourney 等报道的平均出血量 3900 mL 相比，说明腹主动脉球囊阻断技术在控制术中出血方面有良好的效果。此外，对行全骶骨切除术的患者，在术前应建立多个输液通道，在术中实行快速输血；如果出血情况严重，输血超过 4000 mL 以上，则应该另外输入血小板及凝血酶原复合物。

全骶骨切除术后容易出现伤口并发症。其原因有以下几个方面：①肿瘤巨大，术后遗留较大的空腔，容易产生积液，易诱发感染；②常规用钉棒系统重建骶髂关节，增加了感染的风险；③部分患者年龄较大，或合并高血压、糖尿病等慢性病；④部分患者因为肿瘤长期消耗或饮食不佳，营养状况不良；⑤部分患者术前曾行放疗。减少伤口并发症的措施包括：①围手术期通过药物控制好高血压、糖尿病等慢性病；②通过各种方式改善患者的营养状况；③术中放置较粗的引流条，适当延长引流时间；④预防性使用抗生素等。如果已经发生了伤口并发症，一般需对伤口进行清创处理。

内固定失败包括内固定物周围感染、内固定物松动或内固定物断裂。如果出现内固定物周围感染，应及时将内固定物取出，行旷置处理；如果出现内固定物松动、断裂，需综合考虑患者的活动功能、疼痛程度、经济条件等，再决定是否行内固定翻修手术。

行全骶骨切除术时，如果损伤神经根袖，则容易在术后出现脑脊液漏。因此，在术中分离肿瘤时应非常小心，避免损伤神经根袖。如果在术后出现脑脊液漏，可先行保守治疗，一般通过抬高床尾、使用抗生素等措施可以治愈。如果脑脊液漏非常严重，保守治疗无效，或者出现感染，使用抗生素无法控制，在必要的时候需考虑手术干预。

骶骨紧贴直肠后方，如果肿瘤巨大，与直肠粘连紧密，在分离肿瘤时，容易造成直肠损伤。因此在术中应小心分离肿瘤，肿瘤离体需仔细检查有无直肠损伤。如果出现直肠损伤，但未穿透肠壁，可在术中直接缝合损伤的肠壁，术后适当延长患者禁食的时间；如果已经穿透肠壁，一般需行造瘘手术。

3.4.2　肿瘤学预后

骶骨原发性恶性骨肿瘤除尤因肉瘤和骨肉瘤外，往往对化疗和放疗不敏感。因此，治疗高位骶骨恶性肿瘤主要依靠手术切除，而行全骶骨切除术则是为了保证高位骶骨恶性肿瘤获得一个满意的外科边界，减少术后复发率，获得治愈的机会。

2009 年 9 月—2017 年 9 月曾在本中心行全骶骨切除术的 52 例患者中，除了失访的 11 例患者，剩下的 41 例患者中，复发 13 例，复发率为 31.7%，其中患者在随访期间死于肿瘤的复发与转移 8 例。既往文献报道的全骶骨切除术后患者的复发率在 8.0%～57.1% 之间。2000 年，Wuisman 等报道的 9 例全骶骨切除术后患者，平均随访时间为 73 个月，出现复发 4 例，复发率为 44.4%，随访期间 3 例死于肿瘤的复发与转移。2000 年，Miles 等报道了 25 例全骶骨切除术患者，平均随访时间为 16 个月，出现局部复发 2 例，复发率为 8.0%，是至今为止最好的报道结果。2003 年，Doita 等报道了 3 例全骶骨切除后患者，其中死于肿瘤的复发 1 例。2005 年，Dickey 等报道了 5 例全骶骨切除术后患者，平均随访时间为 18 个月，其中复发 2 例，并死于肿瘤的复发与转移，复发率为 40.0%。2008年刘世清等报道了 7 例全骶骨切除术后患者，术后随访 6 ～ 36 个月，出现复发 4 例，复发率为 57.1%，后来均死于肿瘤复发。2014 年，孙伟等报道了 5 例全骶骨切除术后患者，其中出现局部复发 1 例，随访期间均带瘤生存，复发率为20.0%。全骶骨切除术理论上有良好的肿瘤边界，但复发率仍然很高，究其原因，一方面可能是肿瘤切除过程中术野有污染或在正常组织内存在卫星灶，未真正完全清除肿瘤；另一方面可能与肿瘤恶性程度较高、侵袭性强有关。

3.4.3　神经功能结局

对于高位骶骨恶性肿瘤，为获得一个满意的外科边界而进行全骶骨切除术，在术中会切除双侧 S1 及以下神经，因此无可避免地会丧失双侧 S1 及以下神经的功能，造成严重的下肢运动功能、大小便功能及性功能的损伤。既往文献对不同水平骶骨切除术后的神经功能结局进行了报道。20 世纪 70 年代，Gunterberg 等对骶骨肿瘤切除术后的神经功能损伤进行了研究，包括大小便功能和性功能的研究，这被认为是这一领域的第一次系统研究。之后的一系列研究认为，保留 S2及以上神经能够让患者保留一定的大小便功能和性功能以具备基本的日常生活能力，而保留双侧 S3 及以上神经的患者，其下肢运动功能和感觉、大小便功能、性功能及其他日常生活能力几乎不受影响。

然而，长期以来骶骨肿瘤术后神经功能的评估缺乏一个广泛认同的标准，大多数研究仅仅使用正常或异常来描述患者的功能状态，无法准确反映患者术后的神经功能结局。1997 年 Biagini 等提出了一个评分系统，对这个领域的发展做出积极的贡献，但这个评分系统具有一定的局限性，还不足以准确地描述骶骨切除术后患者的神经功能结局。2016 年，黄林等在 Biagini 的评分系统的基础上进行了拓展，提出了一个新的评分系统，其内容更加充分翔实，区分度更高，通过这个系统可以得到一个 0 ～ 27 分的总分，对神经功能进行定量分析，能更加准确地描述骶骨肿瘤术后患者的神经功能状态。本研究采用了黄林等建立的骶骨切除术后神经功能评分系统对全骶骨切除术后患者的神经功能结局进行评估。

从本研究的结果可以看到，全骶骨切除术对患者的神经功能产生了非常显著的影响。本研究首次引用黄林等建立的骶骨切除术后神经功能评分系统进行评价，并且是首次专门针对全骶骨切除术后患者的神经功能结局进行了定量分析。通过研究患者神经功能评分的得分，本研究对全骶骨切除术后患者的神经功能结局有了更深的认识，并可以对全骶骨切除术后患者的神经功能进行基本的预期。在下肢活动方面，患者在行走时需要借助拐杖、助步器等外部支持；在疼痛方面，患者会出现需要镇痛药控制的疼痛或轻度疼痛；在会阴感觉方面，患者会出现影响日常生活的会阴感觉，如麻木或过敏；在排尿困难方面，患者可能会出现轻度的排尿困难，也可能需要用手挤压腹部辅助排尿；在尿失禁方面，患者会出现频繁漏尿，需要使用尿布；在膀胱感觉方面，患者排尿有时会丧失膀胱的感觉；在便秘方面，患者有中度的便秘，常常需要进行灌肠或者导泄；在大便失禁方面，患者可能会偶尔失禁，也可能频繁失禁；在直肠感觉方面，患者有时在排便时会丧失直肠感觉。

本研究的数据，可以让临床工作者获得对全骶骨切除术后的神经功能较为准确的预期，对患者术后的大小便功能和下肢功能进行相对合理的判断，以便更好地衡量手术的成本与获益，从而更好地指导医疗决策、管理患者围手术期的预期以及促进患者康复。

3.4.4　健康相关生命质量

现代医学的共识要求对骶骨恶性肿瘤行根治性整块切除以达到最好的局部控制效果，然而对于高位骶骨恶性肿瘤的患者而言，为了获得满意的肿瘤学边界而行全骶骨切除术后，必然丢失 S5 及以下神经的功能，从而对患者的生命质量产生极大的影响。以往研究骶骨肿瘤预后的文献往往局限于肿瘤学预后和神经功能结局，很少针对患者术后的健康相关生命质量进行研究，从而无法评估肿瘤及手术对患者心理健康及社会功能等方面的影响，无法全面评估患者的健康结局。

2016 年，Phukan 等使用患者 PROMIS 评估系统对 33 例不同切除水平的骶骨切除术后患者进行了健康相关生命质量的评估，平均随访时间 41 个月，发现骶骨切除术的截骨水平越高，术后患者的健康相关生命质量越低。这应该是国际上第一次对骶骨肿瘤术后患者的生命质量进行系统的评估。国内还没有发现关于这方面的报道。由于高位骶骨肿瘤发病率很低，且全骶骨切除术手术难度极大，因此既往文献报道的全骶骨切除术例数往往较少。本研究评价了 33 例全骶骨切除术后患者的健康相关生命质量，在全骶骨切除术后患者的例数上居于国际首位。

笔者在选择研究全骶骨切除术后患者的健康相关生命质量的工具时，查阅了相关文献，发现仅有 Phukan 等使用 PROMIS 系统对骶骨肿瘤术后的患者进行了健康相关生命质量的评估。因此，笔者参考了脊柱肿瘤患者术后的健康相关生命质量研究，发现相关学者往往使用各种健康相关生命质量量表对患者进行评估，这些量表包括 SF-36 量表、PROMIS 系统、EQ-5D 量表、ODI 指数、KPS 评分、ECOG 量表等。这些评价工具具有非常重要的参考价值，但本研究并不直接套用这些量表。由于这些量表都是由不同国家的学者进行研制的，在研制过程中这些学者考虑的是本国的文化背景和其特定人群的健康水平，因此这些量表不一定适用于中国的文化背景和中国普通人群的健康水平。为了确保研究结果的准确性，本研究在使用国外的生命质量量表之前，需要对量表进行汉语翻译，并针对国内人群进行性能测试，制订中国普通人群的常模。通过查阅中文文献，笔者发现 SF-36 v2 量表针对中国人群进行的性能测试和常模制订，可直接应用于中国患者的临床研究。SF-36 v2 量表一共有 36 个问题，从生理功能、生理职能、躯体疼痛、总体健康、活力、社会功能、情感职能以及精神健康等 8 个方面全面概括了被调查者的生存质量，笔者认为其问题的内容非常适合用于评价全骶骨切除术后患者的健康相关生命质量评估，因此最终选定了 SF-36 v2 量表。

本研究通过 SF-36 v2 量表评估了全骶骨切除术后患者的健康相关生命质量，与中国普通人群常模进行对比后，发现全骶骨切除术后患者的生理健康总分和心理健康总分均有明显的下降，且生理健康总分的下降要比心理健康总分的下降更加明显，这与 2016 年 Phukan 等的报道相一致。本研究探索了全骶骨切除术后患者健康相关生命质量的影响因素，发现神经功能评分总分和生理健康总分以及心理健康总分均存在相关性，神经功能评分总分和生理健康总分之间的相关性要比其与心理健康总分之间的相关性更明显。这是可以理解的，因为全骶骨切除术让患者丧失了 S5 及以下神经的功能，能直接影响患者的生理健康，但对患者心理健康的影响却是间接的。本研究发现，患者的年龄、性别、社会经济地位评分、病理类型、出血量、手术并发症、手术入路等因素对患者的健康相关生命质量的影响没有统计学差异，这可能与本研究的病例数太少有关，之后随着全骶骨切除术后患者例数的增加，我们或许能有新的发现。

3.4.5　本研究的局限性

首先，本研究的样本量比较小，仅有 33 例。这是在研究罕见疾病时的一个无法避免的难题。尽管与既有文献相比，本研究中全骶骨切除术后患者例数已居于首位，但样本量的局限性仍然影响了本研究结论的准确性。比如，本研究中尝试探索全骶骨切除术后患者健康相关生命质量的影响因素，但可能样本量太小，导致患者的年龄、性别、社会经济地位评分、病理类型、出血量、手术并发症、手术入路等因素造成的影响缺乏统计学意义。将来随着病例数的增加，我们将会得出更准确的结论，也有可能获得新的发现。

其次，本研究缺乏患者术前神经功能状态和健康相关生命质量的数据。患者在术前的神经功能状态可能与健康人群一致，也可能低于健康人群；患者在术前的健康相关生命质量则可能高于、等于或低于一般人群，因为健康相关生命质量与患者的主观感受联系密切。由于无法进行手术前后的比较，因此无法准确地评估肿瘤及全骶骨切除术对患者神经功能和健康相关生命质量的影响。

此外，本研究 33 例患者的随访时间是不一致的（4～93 个月），可能影响本研究结论的准确性。一方面，随访时间太短使本研究缺乏足够的数据分析患者的肿瘤学预后，难以准确评估患者远期的生存状况。另一方面，患者的神经功能结局和健康相关生命质量可能会随着随访时间的变化而变化。Moran 等发现在术后12 个月的随访过程中，骶骨切除术后患者的神经功能状态有显著的变化：排尿功能在术后 3 个月内有较大变化，下肢功能在术后 6 个月有较大变化，而排便功能则没有明显随时间的延长而改变的趋势。另外，有文献报道，骶骨切除术后患者需要 6 个月的时间恢复下肢活动和大小便功能。以后随着病例的增加和随访时间的延长，我们将关注随访时间对全骶骨切除术后患者神经功能结局和健康相关生命质量的影响。

最后，由于缺乏合适的评估全骶骨切除术后性功能水平的工具，本研究并未对患者的性功能进行评估。这个领域还需要更多相关学者的关注和参与。如果将来有合适的评价体系，我们会对患者术后的性功能进行更多的探索。

4　全骶骨切除术后患者体验的定性分析

4.1　前言

全骶骨切除术是高位骶骨恶性肿瘤主要的治疗方式，由于术中切断了 S5 及以下神经，术后患者长期处于下肢功能、大小便功能和性功能明显受损的病态情况，严重影响了患者的活动能力和日常生活能力。这种情况相对其他肿瘤而言是非常独特的。

既往文献还没有针对全骶骨切除术后患者的长期生活体验进行报道。2010年，Davidge 等采用半结构化访谈的方法对 12 例骶骨切除术后患者的体验进行了研究，但可惜的是其中并没有全骶骨切除术后的病例。本研究首次采用定性分析的方法研究全骶骨切除术后患者的生活及情感体验。

定性分析的方法能够深入探讨患者的个人体验，有利于评估疾病对患者个人生活和情感体验的影响。本研究将采取半结构化访谈这种定性分析的方法研究全骶骨切除术后患者的生活体验。

研究患者术后的生活体验及情感体验，能够让医生和其他医疗工作人员更好地理解患者在全骶骨切除术后的生理、心理、社会和情感经历，有利于外科医生和其他保健工作者更好地指导手术决策，管理患者围手术期的期望，并更好地协助患者康复。

4.2　研究对象和研究方法

4.2.1　研究对象

与第 2 部分 3.2.1 研究的患者一致，其一般资料可参见第 2 部分 3.2 的研究对象的内容。

4.2.2　研究方法

本研究采取定性分析的方法研究全骶骨切除术后患者的生活体验，其理论基础是扎根理论。扎根理论的宗旨是在经验资料的基础上建立理论，即研究者在研究开始之前一般没有理论假设，直接从实际观察入手，将原始资料进行整理、分析、比较、归纳、概括，然后上升到系统的理论。本研究没有对全骶骨切除术后患者的生活体验进行假设，而是先对患者进行半结构化访谈，在访谈中收集关于他们生活体验的资料，然后将这些资料进行分类、比较、整合，从而得出研究结果。

定性分析的基本方法包括观察、访谈、案例研究等。本研究使用的半结构化访谈属于访谈中的一种，即按照一个粗线条式的提纲对患者进行访谈，但访谈时提问的方式和顺序、访谈对象回答的方式、访谈记录的方式和访谈的时间、地点等均可由访谈者灵活处理。

本研究中半结构化访谈的提纲是由数位外科医生和一位心理医生共同制订的。外科医生提出感兴趣的方向并初步制订访谈的提纲，然后由心理医生进行审查和调整。本研究主要围绕以下 8 个主题进行半结构化访谈：①日常生活能力；②社会交际情况；③学习或工作情况；④对家庭的影响；⑤对造瘘手术的接受程度；⑥对远期康复指导的需求；⑦对住院期间医疗服务的满意度；⑧对治疗结局的满意度。

本研究由一位外科医生进行访谈，由一位心理医生进行访谈的监督和指导。访谈者与患者约定好时间，通过电话访谈的方式，对患者进行半结构化访谈，访谈时进行即时录音，访谈结束后对录音内容进行记录和整理。本研究从 2017 年 11 月 1 日开始，至 2018 年 1 月 31 日结束，为期 3 个月。平均访谈时间为 26 分钟（范围 17 ～ 63 分钟）。

4.3　研究结果

4.3.1　日常生活能力

在与患者进行访谈时，主要通过吃饭、洗澡、大小便以及活动能力几个方面研究患者的日常生活能力。通过对访谈资料的整理，对患者进行了简单的分类。其中 11 例患者具有接近常人的日常生活能力，能够做到生活自理，日常生活不需要依赖他人。而另外 22 例患者则无法做到生活自理，无法离开他人的帮助。他们无法生活自理的原因有以下几个方面：①缺乏行走能力，有的患者长期卧床，或者必须在家人搀扶下才能偶尔行走；②无法大幅度弯腰或下蹲，因此做某些事情如穿裤子等有很大的难度；③有严重的大小便功能障碍，部分患者需要家人帮忙用手协助排便，部分行结肠造瘘或输尿管造瘘的患者需要家人协助换袋。表 4.1 列举了比较具有代表意义的患者陈述。

表 4.1　患者的日常生活能力情况

分类	患者陈述
需要他人帮助 （n=22）	走路离不开扶架，手够不着脚，自己穿不了裤子和袜子，剪不了趾甲，起床时还得爱人扶我一把
	除了吃饭，其他事情包括穿裤子、洗澡都得家人帮着我
	不能完全自理，很多事情都需要家人帮忙，走路得家人扶着，换尿袋也得家人帮我换
	我离不开我妈妈，我可以自己穿裤子、鞋子、刷牙、吃饭，但是洗澡、大小便都需要妈妈帮忙
	我下不了床，走不了路，什么事情都要家人帮我
完全生活自理 （n=11）	生活都能自理，能走能挪，不需要别人帮忙
	我完全能够自己解决，不需要依靠他人

4.3.2　社会交际情况

在 33 例患者中，共有 28 例患者自诉在进行全骶骨切除术后他们的社会交际活动相比术前明显减少。他们有的长期卧床，无法下地；有的虽然可以行走，但行走能力不强，出门比较困难；有的则因为严重的大小便失禁问题不方便参加活动；有的则是容易疲劳，没有精力参与社会交际。另外 5 例患者自诉与术前相比他们的社会交际情况基本正常，这些患者术后功能恢复得非常好，特别是下肢活动功能，而且他们非常乐观，有积极的生活态度，不把自己当作病人，而是以正常人的心态面对生活。表 4.2 列举了具有代表意义的患者陈述。

表 4.2　患者的社会交际情况

分类	患者陈述
社会交际明显减少 （n=28）	我整天躺在床上，下不了地，根本出不了门
	我平时都只能在家里走动，走不远，不方便出去走动
	因为尿失禁情况太严重了，一不小心就会漏尿，出去很不方便，所以比较少出去和朋友玩
	做完手术以后体力就没之前那么好了，容易疲劳，就算朋友约我出去，我也很少去了

续表

分类	患者陈述
基本正常 （*n*=5）	我经常自己开车，和朋友一块外出旅游，或者和朋友一起唱歌，去寺庙拜佛
	隔三岔五出去串串门，上亲戚家走走都没问题
	经常有亲朋好友来看我，陪我聊天，让我觉得家里一直都挺热闹的

4.3.3　学习或工作情况

在 33 例患者中，一共有 28 例患者在术后未能恢复至正常的学习或工作。其主要原因还是受限于他们的下肢活动能力，他们没有足够的能力胜任工作岗位的要求，尤其是体力劳动者。有的患者家属担心患者身体情况，不允许患者出去工作。其中 2 例患者术前是学生，术后均因为身体原因未能继续上学。这种情况对患者的影响其实是很大的。对于学生而言，不能继续上学，对其未来的人生发展会产生非常巨大的影响。对于年富力强、正处于工作年龄的患者来说，不能工作意味着家庭少了 1 个重要的经济来源。仅有 5 例患者可以正常工作，其中，2 例是企业管理人员，1 例是医生，1 例是公务员，1 例是收银员，在工作时基本不会有太多的体力劳动，因此，他们在恢复了一定的下肢活动能力后，很快回到了工作岗位。表 4.3 列举了具有代表意义的患者陈述。

表 4.3　患者的学习或工作情况

分类	患者陈述
无法上学或工作 （*n*=28）	起不来，整天躺在床上，什么都做不了
	生病前我和老伴开店卖家电，做完手术后就干不了了，老伴还要照顾我，只能把店关了
	我原来是修车的，做完手术后身体不行了，吃不消
	我其实想出去干点零活的，但是家人不让我去，怕出问题，我只能在家里做些力所能及的家务活
	我生病后就休学了，做完手术后一直没能上学，因为我行动不方便，需要家人照顾，在学校没法照顾自己，我特别羡慕那些能正常上学的同学
正常工作 （*n*=5）	手术后我恢复得很好，很快就回到了原来的工作岗位，基本对工作生活没有太大影响
	我恢复得不错，现在已经回医院上班了
	我在家附近的商店当收银员，工作上倒不是特别吃力

4.3.4　对家庭的影响

在 33 例患者中，有 29 例患者认为肿瘤及手术治疗对家庭产生了非常大的影响。有的患者家庭经济水平不高，难以承受高昂的手术费用；有的患者在术后丧失了日常生活能力，离不开家人的照顾，严重影响了家人的工作和生活。患者在承受病痛的折磨时，家人一般与患者感同身受。但是通过访谈我们发现了2个特殊的例子：1例是由于家人没有精力照顾，被迫将患者送至养老院；另1例是患者的丈夫不愿照顾患者，强行与患者离婚，患者只能寻求年老的父母帮忙照顾。由此可见，肿瘤以及手术不仅影响患者个人，还对患者的家庭产生巨大的打击，甚至引发家庭破裂。仅有4例患者认为肿瘤及手术没有对其家庭产生太大的影响。这4例患者中有3例患者可以正常工作，有1例患者已经退休，他们都有良好的日常生活能力，因而不需要家人特别照顾。当然他们并不否认手术期间以及术后一段时间对家庭产生的影响，只是他们目前恢复良好，家庭已经回到正轨，肿瘤及手术所产生的影响已经基本远去。表4.4列举了具有代表意义的患者陈述。

表4.4　全骶骨切除术对患者家庭的影响

分类	患者陈述
影响很大 （n=29）	经济负担太大了，做手术花了20多万，我们农村家庭真的难以承受
	妈妈为了照顾我辞掉了工作，爸爸也为了我来回奔波，严重影响了工作
	我爱人为了照顾我，需要经常请假，太影响工作了
	全家的精力都在我身上，我疼痛发作的时候，全家的人都围着我转
	我就一个女儿，她又要工作又要照顾孩子，实在没有时间照顾我，只能把我送到养老院去
	做完手术后，婚姻关系不和谐导致离婚
没有太大影响 （n=4）	我现在工作都正常，对家庭基本没什么影响，跟生病前差不多
	对整个家庭影响不大，如果有什么不舒服也是我自己去面对这个事情，平时也不需要家人照顾我

4.3.5　对造瘘手术的接受程度

在33例患者中，有30例患者表示不愿意接受造瘘手术，其中有1例由于术中损伤直肠已行结肠造瘘，自述造瘘袋不方便处理。另外29例患者不愿意接受造瘘手术的原因有以下几点：①大小便功能恢复良好，认为没有必要；②大小便功能不算太好，表示可以适应目前的状况；③认为大小便功能还有恢复的机会；④认为造瘘手术影响美观，对以后的婚姻可能产生影响；⑤还有的患者肿瘤复发问题未能得到解决，暂不考虑这个问题。仅有3例患者表示愿意接受造瘘手术，其中1例在术中损伤肠道已行造瘘手术，认为造瘘袋护理还算方便，不影响生活；1例患者无法忍受长期留置尿管的痛苦，于外院行输尿管造瘘手术，对现状表示满意；1例患者无法接受长期尿失禁的现状，希望通过造瘘手术解决这个问题。表4.5列举了具有代表意义的患者陈述。

表 4.5　患者对造瘘手术的接受程度

分类	患者陈述
不愿意接受（n=30）	我大小便功能恢复得挺好的，没有做手术的必要
	虽然现在大小便确实不太方便，但也还能凑合，不想再折腾了
	刚做完手术的时候我大小便完全失禁，现在已经恢复了一点，基本上能够控制了，最好还是不要做那个手术，心理上接受不了
	在肚子上打个洞太不美观了，我还年轻，还没有结婚，不能接受这种事情
	太不方便了，我自己换不了，都是我家人帮我更换造瘘袋
	我现在肿瘤复发的问题都不能解决，哪有心思考虑这个问题
愿意接受（n=3）	我现在整天尿裤子，非常不方便，如果能解决失禁的问题，也是可以接受的
	我基本上能自己处理造瘘袋，弄得比较干净，没有什么异味
	手术之后因为尿不出来，一直要插尿管，实在是太痛苦了，后来我就在我们附近的医院做了输尿管造瘘手术，现在觉得挺好的

4.3.6　对远期康复指导的需求

参与访谈的 33 例患者对远期康复指导均有不同程度的需求。一般而言，医生在围手术期会反复向患者解释手术带来的获益、可能存在的风险、术后可能出现的结局以及如何进行康复，但是患者在短期内接收了大量的信息，对这些信息的理解无法达到医生的预期，并在出院之后逐渐忘记。全骶骨切除术后患者比较特殊，在出院后的几个月内没有行走的能力，到医院进行复诊非常困难，如果患者出现了新的病情，他们往往不知所措。另外，患者在出院时的下肢功能、大小便功能一般处于低谷，在出院后随着时间的延长会逐渐恢复，但是患者并不清楚他们的功能最终能恢复到什么程度，也不知道他们当前的状态是否正常。因此，有患者希望医生提供一个关于康复指导的文字材料，方便他们随时查看。也有患者与医生通过微信联系，在出现新病情时方便联系。表 4.6 列举了具有代表意义的患者陈述。

表 4.6　患者对远期康复指导的需求

	患者陈述
患者对远期康复指导的需求	医生当时说得挺详细的，我也按照他们说的做了，但我不知道我这个病能恢复成啥样，也不知道我现在的情况是不是正常的
	当时医生对后面怎么恢复说得比较清楚，但主要是口头交代，现在很多都忘了，我希望能有文字说明，说清楚什么时候做什么动作，什么事情不能做等等，方便随时拿出来看看

续表

	患者陈述
患者对远期康复指导的需求	医生有比较详细的指导，而且加了我的微信，我对我的病情有什么疑问的话会通过微信咨询他
	我当时不知道如何翻身以及需要注意什么，但是医生说我怎么舒服怎么来，没有告诉我具体的指导，我就自己折腾了，不知道做得对不对

4.3.7 对住院期间医疗服务的满意度

全骶骨切除术后患者的住院时间一般比较长，接近1个月。我们的医护团队在做手术之前会对患者进行相关的训练，在手术之后指导患者进行肢体训练，协助患者翻身和大小便等，这种训练会一直持续到患者出院，因此，患者和我们的医护团队在住院期间有非常密切的互动交流。从访谈结果来看，有32例患者对我们医护团队给予了积极的评价，只有1例患者，因为术中损伤了肠道，术后出现了严重的感染，后来进行了2次清创手术和1次内固定取出手术，患者因此非常痛苦，手术也给患者家属带来了沉重的经济负担，所以对我们医护团队表示不满。表4.7列举了具有代表意义的患者陈述。

表4.7 患者对住院期间医疗服务的评价

分类	患者陈述
满意 (*n*=32)	医生和护士都特别好、非常负责，我在医院的时候曾经非常绝望，连续哭了好几天，妈妈都劝不住我，最后还是护士来安慰我，给我做思想工作
	医生技术高超，态度和蔼，工作认真细心，我在看护士换药的时候，觉得就像看一门艺术
	医生、护士技术不错，非常负责任，对患者态度也好
不满意 (*n*=1)	手术时出现严重感染，害我多做了几次手术，遭了很大的罪，多花了很多钱

4.3.8 对治疗结局的满意度

本研究在访谈的最后询问了患者对治疗结局的满意度。大部分患者都对治疗结局表示满意。尽管有部分患者术后功能恢复不佳，但是他们认为手术治疗帮助他们治愈了肿瘤，挽救了生命，并对我们表示了感谢。不过还是有10例患者对治疗结局表示不满，其中5例肿瘤复发的患者均无法接受自己的结局，表示非常无奈；另外5例患者则因为术后下肢活动、大小便功能恢复不佳或者顽固性的疼痛而无法接受现状。表4.8列举了具有代表意义的患者陈述。

表 4.8　患者对治疗结局的满意度

分类	患者陈述
满意 （n=23）	非常感谢医生，手术做得很好，我恢复得也很好，对现在的情况很满意
	我在来你们医院之前，别的医院都说做完这个手术基本上不可能站起来，而且大小便一定会失禁，但是现在我的情况比我想象的要好得多，感觉比较满意
	我这是恶性肿瘤，现在没死没残废，还能走能摆，感觉相当满意
	虽然现在生活很不方便，但是至少你们帮我把肿瘤治好，挽救了我的生命，我非常感谢你们
不满意 （n=10）	肯定不满意啊，做完以后很快就复发了，现在手术也做不了了，大夫说放疗、化疗都没用，彻底没办法了
	不满意，因为行走很不方便，还有小便失禁，严重影响了我的生活
	不满意，做完手术后腿又疼又麻，吃止疼药也不管用，真是太痛苦了
	非常后悔，我无法接受现在这么不好的情况，给爱人、儿女带来了很大的负担，而且治病花了很多钱，我宁愿不治病，把钱留给我的儿子和孙子

4.4　讨论

本研究首次通过半结构化访谈的方式对全骶骨切除术后患者的体验进行定性分析，既往文献还没有过类似的报道。2010 年，Davidge 等采用半结构化访谈的方法对 12 例骶骨切除术后患者的体验进行了研究，但可惜的是其中并没有全骶骨切除术后的病例。

定性分析区别于定量分析，多见于社会科学领域的研究，在临床和生物医学领域比较少见，但定性分析在临床和生物医学领域是不可或缺的组成部分，一方面它可以让我们对定量研究无能为力的领域进行研究，另一方面它是陌生领域进行定量分析的前期条件。本研究的内容是全骶骨切除术对患者体验的影响，既往还未有关于这方面的研究报道，也没有进行定量分析的工具，因此有必要使用定性分析的方法。通过查阅文献，我们发现骨肿瘤领域也有一些定性分析的报道：2006 年，Wright 等用定性分析的方法研究了直肠癌患者行扩大的骨盆切除术后的体验；2010 年，Henderson 等用定性分析的方法研究了使用可延长假体行保肢手术的骨肉瘤儿童患者的情感接受程度；2015 年，Fauske 等对骨盆肿瘤、肢体骨肉瘤对患者生活的影响进行了定性分析。这些都证明了定性分析研究方法所具有的价值。

从本研究的结果可以看到，进行全骶骨切除术的患者中，除了小部分功能恢复非常顺利的患者可以回到接近正常的生活状态，大部分患者在日常生活能力、社会交际情况、学习和工作方面都受到非常显著的负面影响，并且也极大地影响了他们的家庭。在访谈中本研究发现，对患者生活影响最大的因素是下肢活动能力，它直接影响了患者的日常生活能力、社会交际能力，决定了患者能否继续上学或者工作，并进一步对家庭产生影响。疼痛和大小便功能障碍也是影响患者生活体验的重要因素。

全骶骨切除术后患者功能恢复的时间较长，且患者的康复非常复杂，需要非常专业的指导，包括下肢功能的训练、大小便的控制、疼痛的控制等。然而，目前患者康复治疗的现状并不乐观。患者在出院后，基本住在家里，依靠家属的协助进行康复。一方面患者及其家属往往缺乏足够的专业知识，难以进行真正有效的功能训练，另一方面患者家属可能也没有足够的精力帮助患者。这些都不利于患者的功能康复。有患者提出，希望可以获得关于康复训练的文字资料或者医生的联系方式以便随时咨询。这其实提示医生，除了在围手术期，在长期的随访过程中对患者及其家属进行医学教育和康复指导也是非常有必要的。医生可以给患者提供康复指导的文字资料，但这不一定能满足所有患者的需要，因为每一位患者都可能会有独特的病情变化。将联系方式留给每一位患者是不现实的，这会耽误医生的正常工作。或许可以寄希望于建立一个专门的康复机构，对全骶骨切除术后的患者进行专业的术后康复，只是目前受限于现实的因素还无法实现，但这无疑是有效解决这个难题的一个方向。

对于高位骶骨肿瘤患者是否应该同期行造瘘手术，目前国际上还没有统一的意见，往往由外科医生进行决定。2016 年，Phukan 等发现行结肠造瘘术并不能提高骶骨切除术后患者的整体生活质量。在我国，除非患者要求或者术中出现了肠道损伤，否则一般不会同期行结肠造瘘手术。2014 年，孙伟等报道了 1 例术中出现肠道损伤并行结肠造瘘手术的全骶骨切除患者，在术后 3 个月又做了造口还纳。本研究访谈的结果发现，大部分患者不愿意接受造瘘手术。随着术后时间的延长和患者自身的适应，全骶骨切除术后患者的大小便功能往往有不同程度的恢复，本研究的大多数患者都能适应大小便功能的现状。因此，笔者认为，没有必要在行全骶骨切除术时同期行造瘘手术，可以给患者一个恢复大小便功能的机会，如果后期患者大小便功能恢复不佳，无法接受大小便功能的状态，可以二期行造瘘手术。

本研究采用半结构化访谈的方式，从患者的角度阐释了全骶骨切除术对患者的神经功能和远期生活体验产生的影响，具有独特的价值。它让医生通过患者的切身体验，更好地理解患者在全骶骨切除术后的生理、心理、社会和情感经历，从而有利于外科医生和其他保健工作者更好地指导手术决策，管理患者围手术期的期望，并更好地协助患者康复。

第 3 部分　结论和展望

1　主要结论

（1）全骶骨切除术治疗高位骶骨恶性肿瘤可以获得满意的肿瘤学切除边界，肿瘤学预后可以令人接受，但是手术并发症发生率较高，造成患者严重的神经功能损伤。

（2）全骶骨切除术严重损害了患者的健康相关生命质量，总体上对生理健康的影响程度大于心理健康的影响程度。患者神经功能结局与健康相关生命质量有明显的正相关，而年龄、性别、社会经济地位评分、病理类型、出血量、手术并发症、手术入路因素对健康相关生命质量的影响没有统计学差异。

（3）用定性分析的方法深入了解了全骶骨切除术后患者的生理、心理、社会和情感体验，证实全骶骨切除术对患者及其家庭的生活造成了非常严重的影响。患者的术后康复需要更多的指导。且患者基本上不愿意接受造瘘手术，没有必要同期行造瘘手术。

（4）全骶骨切除术需严格把握适应证，并向患者充分告知手术的获益和潜在的风险，以便更好地进行手术决策，管理患者围手术期的预期，帮助患者康复。

2　创新点

（1）本研究中全骶骨切除术后患者的样本量高于以往所有相关文献的报道，为全骶骨切除术后患者的外科治疗结局、肿瘤学预后提供了更大样本的数据。

（2）首次使用黄林等建立的骶骨切除术后神经功能评分系统，专门针对全骶骨切除术后患者的神经功能结局进行了定量的评估。

（3）在国内首次对全骶骨切除术后的健康相关生命质量进行了评估。

（4）首次使用定性分析的方法研究了全骶骨切除术后患者的生活和情感体验。

（5）首次同时使用神经功能评分系统、健康相关生命质量量表和定性分析等方法，对全骶骨切除术后患者的外科治疗结局、健康相关生命质量以及生活和情感体验进行了研究，从不同的角度全面深入分析全骶骨切除术后患者的预后情况。

3 局限性

（1）样本量较小，尽管本研究的样本量超过了既往相关文献的报道，但其局限性仍然影响了本研究结论的准确性。今后，随着病例的增加，我们将会得出更加详细、准确的结论。

（2）本研究缺乏患者术前神经功能状态和健康相关生命质量的数据，无法进行手术前后的比较，从而无法准确地评估肿瘤及全骶骨切除术对患者神经功能和健康相关生命质量的影响。因此，有必要进行一个前瞻性的研究，将患者手术前后的数据进行对比，以便更准确地评价手术对神经功能和健康相关生命质量的影响。

（3）本研究中33例患者的随访时间是不一致的，而患者术后功能恢复与随访时间长短有一定关系，这可能影响本研究结论的准确性。因此，我们有必要对患者进行更长时间的随访，以分析患者的神经功能和健康相关生命质量随着时间的延长而产生的改变，得出更准确的结论。

（4）由于缺乏合适的评估全骶骨切除术后性功能水平的工具，本研究并未对患者术后的性功能进行评估。这个领域还需要更多相关学者的关注和参与。如果将来有合适的评价体系，我们会对患者术后的性功能进行更多的探索。

参考文献

—◆◆◆◆◆—

［1］KAYANI B，SEWELL M D，HANNA S A，et al. Prognostic Factors in the Operative Management of Dedifferentiated Sacral Chordomas ［J］. Neurosurgery，2014，75（3）：269-275.

［2］KAYANI B，SEWELL M D，TAN K A，et al. Prognostic Factors in the Operative Management of Sacral Chordomas ［J］. World Neurosurg，2015，84（5）：1354-1361.

［3］JI T，GUO W，YANG R，et al. What Are the Conditional Survival and Functional Outcomes After Surgical Treatment of 115 Patients With Sacral Chordoma？［J］. Clin Orthop Relat Res，2017，475（3）：620-630.

［4］VAN WULFFTEN PALTHE O D，HOUDEK M T，ROSE P S，et al. How Does the Level of Nerve Root Resection in En Bloc Sacrectomy Influence Patient-Reported Outcomes？［J］. Clin Orthop Relat Res，2017，475（3）：607-616.

［5］PILLAI S，GOVENDER S. Sacral chordoma：A review of literature ［J］. J Orthop，2018，15（2）：679-684.

［6］CHEN K W，YANG H L，KANDIMALLA Y，et al. Review of current treatment of sacral chordoma ［J］. Orthop Surg，2009，1（3）：238-244.

［7］BRANCO E SILVA M，BRANCO E SILVA M，CONCEIÇÃO MAIA MARTINS S，et al. Analysis of morbidity and mortality in patients with primary bone tumors who underwent sacrectomy：A systematic review ［J］. J Bone Oncol，2022（35）：100445.

［8］FIANI B，RUNNELS J，ROSE A，et al. Clinical manifestations，classification，and surgical management of sacral tumors and the need for personalized approach to sacrectomy ［J］. Surg Neurol Int，2021（12）：209.

［9］ZUCKERMAN S L，LEE S H，CHANG G J，et al. Outcomes of Surgery for Sacral Chordoma and Impact of Complications：A Report of 50 Consecutive Patients with Long-Term Follow-Up ［J］. Global Spine J，2021，11（5）：740-750.

[10] WALCUTT J E，JOHNSON C M，LY Q P，et al. Metastatic Giant Cell Tumor Causing Small Bowel Intussusception on 18 F-FDG PET/CT [J]. Clin Nucl Med，2022，47（11）：963-964.

[11] POTTER G D，MCCLENNAN B L. MALIGNANT GIANT CELL TUMOR OF THE SPHENOID BONE AND ITS DIFFERENTIAL DIAGNOSIS [J]. Cancer，1970，25（1）：167-170.

[12] KATTNER K A，STROINK A，GUPTA K，et al. Giant Cell Tumor of the Sphenoid Bone [J]. Skull Base Surg，1998，8（2）：93-97.

[13] JAMIL O A，LECHPAMMER M，PRASAD S，et al. Giant cell reparative granuloma of the sphenoid：Case report and review of the literature [J]. Surg Neurol Int，2012（3）：140.

[14] NAKAMURA H，MORISAKO H，OHATA H，et al. Pediatric giant cell reparative granuloma of the lower clivus：A case report and review of the literature [J]. J Craniovertebr Junction Spine，2021，12（1）：86-90.

[15] SHRESTHA S，ZHANG J，YAN J，et al. Radiological features of central giant cell granuloma：comparative study of 7 cases and literature review [J]. Dentomaxillofac Radiol，2021，50（5）：20200429.

[16] ZHENG S，ZHOU S，QIAO G，et al. Pirarubicin-based chemotherapy displayed better clinical outcomes and lower toxicity than did doxorubicin-based chemotherapy in the treatment of non-metastatic extremity osteosarcoma [J]. Am J Cancer Res，2014，5（1）：411-422.

[17] YU W，TANG L，LIN F，et al. Pirarubicin versus doxorubicin in neoadjuvant/adjuvant chemotherapy for stage IIB limb high-grade osteosarcoma：Does the analog matter？[J]. Med Oncol，2015，32（1）：307.

[18] KALIFA C，BRUGIÈRES L，LE DELEY M C. Neoadjuvant treatment in osteosarcomas [J]. Bull Cancer，2006，93（11）：1115-1120.

[19] FERRARI S，SMELAND S，MERCURI M，et al. Neoadjuvant Chemotherapy With High-Dose Ifosfamide，High-Dose Methotrexate，Cisplatin，and Doxorubicin for Patients With Localized Osteosarcoma of the Extremity：A Joint Study by the Italian and Scandinavian Sarcoma Groups [J]. J Clin Oncol，2005，23（34）：8845-8852.

［20］MACIEJCZAK A，GASIK R，KOTRYCH D，et al. Spinal tumours：recommendations of the Polish Society of Spine Surgery，the Polish Society of Oncology，the Polish Society of Neurosurgeons，the Polish Society of Oncologic Surgery，the Polish Society of Oncologic Radiotherapy，and the Polish Society of Orthopaedics and Traumatology［J］. Eur Spine J，2023，32（4）：1300-1325.

［21］TIAN Z，NIU X，YAO W. Receptor Tyrosine Kinases in Osteosarcoma Treatment：Which Is the Key Target？［J］. Front Oncol，2020（10）：1642.

［22］FLEUREN E D G，VLENTERIE M，VAN DER GRAAF W T A. Recent advances on anti-angiogenic multi-receptor tyrosine kinase inhibitors in osteosarcoma and Ewing sarcoma［J］. Front Oncol，2023（13）：1013359.

［23］WANG Z X，GUO M Y，REN J，et al. Identification of Lysosome-Associated Protein Transmembrane-4 as a Novel Therapeutic Target for Osteosarcoma Treatment［J］. Orthop Surg，2020，12（4）：1253-1260.

［24］ZHANG L，YANG L，XIA Z W，et al. RETRACTED ARTICLE：The role of fibroblast activation protein in progression and development of osteosarcoma cells［J］. Clin Exp Med，2020，20（1）：121-130.

［25］WANG Z X，REN S C，CHANG Z S，et al. Identification of Kinesin Family Member 2A（KIF2A）as a Promising Therapeutic Target for Osteosarcoma［J］. Biomed Res Int，2020（2020）：7102757.

［26］CHOW W A. Chondrosarcoma：biology，genetics，and epigenetics［J］. F1000Res，2018（7）：F1000 Faculty Rev-1826.

［27］GELDERBLOM H，HOGENDOORN P C，DIJKSTRA S D，et al. The Clinical Approach Towards Chondrosarcoma［J］. Oncologist，2008，13（3）：320-329.

［28］MCLOUGHLIN G S，SCIUBBA D M，WOLINSKY J P. Chondroma/Chondrosarcoma of the Spine［J］. Neurosurg Clin N Am，2008，19（1）：57-63.

［29］KATTEPUR A K，JONES R L，GULIA A. Dedifferentiated chondrosarcoma：current standards of care［J］. Future Oncol，2021，17（35）：4983-4991.

［30］AMER K M，MUNN M，CONGIUSTA D，et al. Survival and Prognosis of Chondrosarcoma Subtypes：SEER Database Analysis［J］. J Orthop Res，2020，38（2）：311-319.

［31］KANO H，NIRANJAN A，LUNSFORD L D. Radiosurgery for Chordoma and

Chondrosarcoma [J]. Prog Neurol Surg，2019（34）：207-214.

［32］HEALEY J H，LANE J M. Chondrosarcoma [J]. Clin Orthop Relat Res，1986（204）：119-129.

［33］MIWA S，YAMAMOTO N，HAYASHI K，et al. Therapeutic Targets and Emerging Treatments in Advanced Chondrosarcoma [J]. Int J Mol Sci，2022，23（3）：1096.

［34］TINOCO G，WILKY B A，PAZ-MEJIA A，et al. The Biology and Management of Cartilaginous Tumors：A Role For Targeting Isocitrate Dehydrogenase [J]. Am Soc Clin Oncol Educ Book，2015：e648-655.

［35］UMEZU H，TAMURA M，KOBAYASHI S，et al. Tracheal chondrosarcoma [J]. Gen Thorac Cardiovasc Surg，2008，56（4）：199-202.

［36］BALAMUTH N J，WOMER R B. Ewing's sarcoma [J]. Lancet Oncol，2010，11（2）：184-192.

［37］CHEN C，BORKER R，EWING J，et al. Epidemiology，Treatment Patterns，and Outcomes of Metastatic Soft Tissue Sarcoma in a Community-Based Oncology Network [J]. Sarcoma，2014，2014：145764.

［38］TURAL D，MOLINAS MANDEL N，DERVISOGLU S，et al. Extraskeletal Ewing's Sarcoma Family of Tumors in Adults：Prognostic Factors and Clinical Outcome [J]. Jpn J Clin Oncol，2012，42（5）：420-426.

［39］GRIER H E，KRAILO M D，TARBELL N J，et al. Addition of Ifosfamide and Etoposide to Standard Chemotherapy for Ewing's Sarcoma and Primitive Neuroectodermal Tumor of Bone [J]. N Engl J Med，2003，348（8）：694-701.

［40］GRIER H E. THE EWING FAMILY OF TUMORS：Ewing's Sarcoma and Primitive Neuroectodermal Tumors [J]. Pediatr Clin North Am，1997，44（4）：991-1004.

［41］PAULUSSEN M，CRAFT A W，LEWIS I，et al. Results of the EICESS-92 Study：Two Randomized Trials of Ewing's Sarcoma Treatment—Cyclophosphamide Compared With Ifosfamide in Standard-Risk Patients and Assessment of Benefit of Etoposide Added to Standard Treatment in High-Risk Patients [J]. J Clin Oncol，2008，26（27）：4385-4393.

［42］MOORE D D，HAYDON R C. Ewing's Sarcoma of Bone [J]. Cancer Treat Res，

2014（162）：93-115.

［43］BACCI G，DI FIORE M，RIMONDINI S，et al. Delayed diagnosis and tumor stage in Ewing's sarcoma［J］. Oncol Rep，1999，6（2）：465-466.

［44］VAN DER HEIJDEN L，FARFALLI G L，BALACÓ I，et al. Biology and technology in the surgical treatment of malignant bone tumours in children and adolescents，with a special note on the very young［J］. J Child Orthop，2021，15（4）：322-330.

［45］HUSAIN R，GARCIA R A，HUANG M，et al. Epiphyseal Ewing Sarcoma in a skeletally mature patient：A case report and review of the literature［J］. Radiol Case Rep，2021，16（5）：1191-1197.

［46］KIATISEVI P，PIYASKULKAEW C，KUNAKORNSAWAT S，et al. What Are the Functional Outcomes After Total Sacrectomy Without Spinopelvic Reconstruction?［J］. Clin Orthop Relat Res，2017，475（3）：643-655.

［47］WUISMAN P，LIESHOUT O，SUGIHARA S，et al. Total Sacrectomy and Reconstruction：Oncologic and Functional Outcome［J］. Clin Orthop Relat Res，2000（381）：192-203.

［48］CLARKE M J，DASENBROCK H，BYDON A，et al. Posterior-Only Approach for En Bloc Sacrectomy：Clinical Outcomes in 36 Consecutive Patients［J］. Neurosurgery，2012，71（2）：357-364.

［49］OLERUD C，JONSSON B. Surgical palliation of symptomatic spinal metastases［J］. Acta Orthop Scand，1996，67（5）：513-522.

［50］WALLACE A N，GREENWOOD T J，JENNINGS J W. Radiofrequency ablation and vertebral augmentation for palliation of painful spinal metastases［J］. J Neurooncol，2015，124（1）：111-118.

［51］BILSKY M H. New therapeutics in spine metastases［J］. Expert Rev Neurother，2005，5（6）：831-840.

［52］BARZILAI O，BILSKY M H，LAUFER I. The Role of Minimal Access Surgery in the Treatment of Spinal Metastatic Tumors［J］. Global Spine J，2020，10（2 Suppl）：79S-87S.

［53］GARNON J，MEYLHEUC L，CAZZATO R L，et al. Percutaneous extra-spinal cementoplasty in patients with cancer：A systematic review of procedural details and clinical outcomes [J]. Diagn Interv Imaging, 2019, 100 (12): 743-752.

[54] 郭卫, 徐万鹏, 杨荣利, 等. 骶骨肿瘤的手术治疗 [J]. 中华外科杂志, 2003, 41 (11): 827-831.

[55] CARNESALE P G. Surgery for Bone and Soft-Tissue Tumors [J]. The Journal of Bone and Joint Surgery, 1998, 80 (10): 1564.

[56] RAQUE G H JR, VITAZ T W, SHIELDS C B. Treatment of Neoplastic Diseases of the Sacrum [J]. J Surg Oncol, 2001, 76 (4): 301-307.

[57] DOITA M, HARADA T, IGUCHI T, et al. Total Sacrectomy and Reconstruction for Sacral Tumors [J]. Spine (Phila Pa 1976), 2003, 28 (15): E296-301.

[58] TOMITA K, TSUCHIYA H. Total Sacrectomy and Reconstruction for Huge Sacral Tumors [J]. Spine (Phila Pa 1976), 1990, 15 (11): 1223-1227.

[59] FOURNEY D R, RHINES L D, HENTSCHEL S J, et al. En bloc resection of primary sacral tumors: classification of surgical approaches and outcome [J]. J Neurosurg Spine, 2005, 3 (2): 111-122.

[60] SHIKATA J, YAMAMURO T, KOTOURA Y, et al. Total sacrectomy and reconstruction for primary tumors. Report of two cases [J]. J Bone Joint Surg Am, 1988, 70 (1): 122-125.

[61] 郭卫, 汤小东, 李大森, 等. 全骶骨切除术治疗骶骨多节段恶性肿瘤 [J]. 中国脊柱脊髓杂志, 2010, 20 (6): 472-476.

[62] HSIEH P C, XU R, SCIUBBA D M, et al. Long-Term Clinical Outcomes Following *En Bloc* Resections for Sacral Chordomas and Chondrosarcomas: a series of twenty consecutive patients [J]. Spine (Phila Pa 1976), 2009, 34 (20): 2233-2239.

[63] 孙伟, 陈泉池, 马小军, 等. 单纯后路全骶骨切除治疗骶骨恶性肿瘤 [J]. 中华骨科杂志, 2014, 34 (11): 1097-1102.

[64] SIMPSON A H, PORTER A, DAVIS A, et al. Cephalad sacral resection with a combined extended ilioinguinal and posterior approach [J]. J Bone Joint Surg Am, 1995, 77 (3): 405-411.

[65] 徐万鹏, 宋献文, 乐守玉, 等. 骶骨肿瘤及其外科治疗 (123 例手术分析) [J]. 中华骨科杂志, 1994, 14 (2): 67-71.

[66] 唐顺, 董森, 郭卫, 等. 腹主动脉球囊阻断控制骶骨肿瘤切除术中出血的效果

［J］. 中国脊柱脊髓杂志，2009，19（2）：85-89.

［67］ FELDMAN F，CASARELLA W J，DICK H M，et al. SELECTIVE INTRA-ARTERIAL EMBOLIZATION OF BONE TUMORS* A USEFUL ADJUNCT IN THE MANAGEMENT OF SELECTED LESIONS ［J］. Am J Roentgenol Radium Ther Nucl Med，1975，123（1）：130-139.

［68］ TANG X，GUO W，YANG R，et al. Use of Aortic Balloon Occlusion to Decrease Blood Loss During Sacral Tumor Resection ［J］. J Bone Joint Surg Am，2010，92（8）：1747-1753.

［69］ 李全，蔡郑东. 全骶骨切除术后重建方式 ［J］. 国际骨科学杂志，2006，27（2）：93-95.

［70］ WUISMAN P，LIESHOUT O，VAN DIJK M，et al. Reconstruction After Total *En Bloc* Sacrectomy for Osteosarcoma Using a Custom-Made Prosthesis：A Technical Note ［J］. Spine（Phila Pa 1976），2001，26（4）：431-439.

［71］ GALLIA G L，HAQUE R，GARONZIK I，et al. Spinal pelvic reconstruction after total sacrectomy for en bloc resection of a giant sacral chordoma ［J］. J Neurosurg Spine，2005，3（6）：501-506.

［72］ MILES W K，CHANG D W，KROLL S S，et al. Reconstruction of Large Sacral Defects Following Total Sacrectomy ［J］. Plast Reconstr Surg，2000，105（7）：2387-2394.

［73］ DICKEY I D，JR H R，FUCHS B，et al. Reconstruction after Total Sacrectomy：Early Experience with a New Surgical Technique ［J］. Clin Ortho Relat Res，2005（438）：42-50.

［74］ 刘世清，丁万军，熊文. 高位骶骨肿瘤切除与骶骨重建方式探讨 ［J］. 中国医师进修杂志，2008，31（7）：18-20.

［75］ NAKAI S，YOSHIZAWA H，KOBAYASHI S，et al. Anorectal and Bladder Function After Sacrifice of the Sacral Nerves ［J］. Spine（Phila Pa 1976），2000，25（17）：2234-2239.

［76］ TODD L T JR，YASZEMSKI M J，CURRIER B L，et al. Bowel and Bladder Function After Major Sacral Resection ［J］. Clin Ortho Relat Res，2002（397）：36-39.

［77］ GUO Y，PALMER J L，SHEN L，et al. Bowel and bladder continence，wound healing，and functional outcomes in patients who underwent sacrectomy［J］. J Neurosurg Spine，2005，3（2）：106-110.

［78］HUANG L，GUO W，YANG R，et al. Proposed Scoring System for Evaluating Neurologic Deficit after Sacral Resection：Functional Outcomes of 170 Consecutive Patients［J］. Spine（Phila Pa 1976），2016，41（7）：628-637.

［79］GUNTERBERG B，PETERSÉN I. Sexual Function After Major Resections of the Sacrum With Bilateral or Unilateral Sacrifice of Sacral Nerves［J］. Fertil Steril，1976，27（10）：1146-1153.

［80］GUNTERBERG B，NORLÉN L，STENER B，et al. Neurourologic evaluation after resection of the sacrum［J］. Invest Urol，1975，13（3）：183-188.

［81］ANDREOLI F，BALLONI F，BIGIOTTI A，et al. Anorectal Continence and Bladder Function：Effects of major sacral resection［J］. Dis Colon Rectum，1986，29（10）：647-652.

［82］FUJIMURA Y，MARUIWA H，TAKAHATA T，et al. Neurological evaluation after radical resection of sacral neoplasms［J］. Paraplegia，1994，32（6）：396-406.

［83］HULEN C A，TEMPLE H T，FOX W P，et al. Oncologic and Functional Outcome Following Sacrectomy for Sacral Chordoma［J］. J Bone Joint Surg Am，2006，88（7）：1532-1539.

［84］PURI A，AGARWAL M G，SHAH M，et al. Decision making in primary sacral tumors［J］. Spine J，2009，9（5）：396-403.

［85］BIAGINI R，RUGGIERI P，MERCURI M，et al. Neurologic deficit after resection of the sacrum［J］. Chir Organi Mov，1997，82（4）：357-372.

［86］MORAN D，ZADNIK P L，TAYLOR T，et al. Maintenance of bowel，bladder，and motor functions after sacrectomy［J］. Spine J，2015，15（2）：222-229.

［87］OMRAN A R. A century of epidemiologic transition in the United States［J］. Prev Med，1977，6（1）：30-51.

［88］HAYS R D，ANDERSON R，REVICKI D. Psychometric considerations in evaluating health-related quality of life measures［J］. Qual Life Res，1993，2（6）：441-449.

［89］COX D R，FITZPATRICK R，FLETCHER A E，et al. Quality-of-Life Assessment：

Can We Keep It Simple？［J］. J R Statist Soc，1992，155（3）：353-375.

［90］ CELLA D F，CHERIN E A. Quality of life during and after cancer treatment ［J］. Comprehensive Therapy，1988，14（5）：69-75.

［91］ SCHIPPER H. Guidelines and caveats for quality of life measurement in clinical practice ［J］. Oncology（Willisto Park），1990，4（5）：51-57.

［92］ ELLWOOD P M. SHATTUCK LECTURE—OUTCOMES MANAGEMENT：A Technology of Patient Experience ［J］. N Eng J Med，1988，318（23）：1549-1556.

［93］ GEIGLE R，JONES S B. Outcomes measurement：a report from the front ［J］. Inquiry，1990，27（1）：7-13.

［94］ TILL J E，OSOBA D，PATER J L，et al. Research on health-related quality of life：dissemination into practical applications ［J］. Qual Life Res，1994，3（4）：279-283.

［95］ 李鲁. 社会医学 ［M］. 3 版. 北京：人民卫生出版社，2007：88-137.

［96］ PHUKAN R，HERZOG T，BOLAND P J，et al. How Does the Level of Sacral Resection for Primary Malignant Bone Tumors Affect Physical and Mental Health，Pain，Mobility，Incontinence，and Sexual Function？［J］. Clin Orthop Relat Res，2016，474（3）：687-696.

［97］ CHAREST-MORIN R，DEA N，FISHER C G. Health-Related Quality of Life After Spine Surgery for Primary Bone Tumour ［J］. Curr Treat Options Oncol，2016，17（2）：1-12.

［98］ KATO S，MURAKAMI H，DEMURA S，et al. More Than 10-Year Follow-Up After Total En Bloc Spondylectomy for Spinal Tumors ［J］. Ann Surg Oncol，2014，21（4）：1330-1336.

［99］ LILJENQVIST U，LERNER T，HALM H，et al. En bloc spondylectomy in malignant tumors of the spine ［J］. Eur Spine J，2008，17（4）：600-609.

［100］ MAZEL C，OWONA P，COGAN A，et al. Long-term quality of life after en-bloc vertebrectomy：25 patients followed up for 9 years ［J］. Orthop Traumatol Surg Res，2014，100（1）：119-126.

［101］ COLMAN M W，KARIM S M，LOZANOCALDERON S A，et al. Quality of life after en bloc resection of tumors in the mobile spine［J］. Spine J，2015，15（8）：

1728-1737.

［102］FAIRBANK J C, PYNSENT P B. The Oswestry Disability Index ［J］. Spine （Phila
Pa 1976）, 2000, 25 （22）: 2940-2952.

［103］SCHAG C C, HEINRICH R L, GANZ P A. Karnofsky performance status revisited:
reliability, validity, and guidelines ［J］. J Clin Oncol, 1984, 2 （3）: 187-193.

［104］OKEN M M, CREECH R H, TORMEY D C, et al. Toxicity and response criteria
of the Eastern Cooperative Oncology Group ［J］. Am J Clin Oncol, 1982, 5 （6）:
649-655.

［105］GANDEK B, WARE J E JR. Methods for Validating and Norming Translations of
Health Status Questionnaires: the IQOLA Project approach. International Quality
of Life Assessment ［J］. J Clin Epidemiol, 1998, 51 （11）: 953-959.

［106］GUILLEMIN F, BOMBARDIER C, BEATON D. Cross-cultural adaptation of
health-related quality of life measures: Literature review and proposed guidelines
［J］. J Clin Epidemiol, 1993, 46 （12）: 1417-1432.

［107］LI L, Wang HM, Shen Y. Chinese SF-36 Health Survey: translation, cultural
adaptation, validation, and normalisation ［J］. J Epidemiol Community Health,
2003, 57 （4）: 259-263.

［108］DAVIDGE K M, ESKICIOGLU C, LIPA J, et al. Qualitative assessment of
patient experiences following sacrectomy ［J］. J Surg Oncol, 2010, 101 （6）:
447-450.

［109］BARSAN V V, BRICEÑO V, GANDHI M, et al. Long-term follow-up and
pregnancy after complete sacrectomy with lumbopelvic reconstruction: case report
and literature review ［J］. BMC Pregnancy Childbirth, 2016 （16）: 1-6.

［110］POPE C, MAYS N. Qualitative Research: Reaching the parts other methods cannot
reach: an introduction to qualitative methods in health and health services research
［J］. BMJ, 1995, 311 （6996）: 42-45.

［111］FAUSKE L, BRULAND O S, GROV E K, et al. Cured of Primary Bone Cancer,
But at What Cost: A Qualitative Study of Functional Impairment and Lost
Opportunities ［J］. Sarcoma, 2015 （2015）: 484196-484205.

［112］FAUSKE L, LOREM G, GROV E K, et al. Changes in the Body Image of Bone
Sarcoma Survivors Following Surgical Treatment—A Qualitative Study ［J］. J

Surg Oncol，2016，113（2）：229-234.

［113］WARE J E JR. SF-36 Health Survey Update［J］. Spine（Phila Pa 1976），2000，25（24）：3130-3139.

［114］李强. 转型时期的中国社会分层结构［M］. 哈尔滨：黑龙江人民出版社，2002：172-175.

［115］FAUSKE L，BONDEVIK H，BRULAND Ø S，et al. Negative and Positive Consequences of Cancer Treatment Experienced by Long-term Osteosarcoma Survivors：A Qualitative Study［J］. Anticancer Res，2015，35（11）：6081-6090.

［116］HENDERSON E R，PEPPER A M，MARULANDA G A，et al. What is the Emotional Acceptance After Limb Salvage with an Expandable Prosthesis？［J］. Clin Orthop Relat Res，2010，468（11）：2933-2938.

［117］WRIGHT F C，CROOKS D，FITCH M，et al. Qualitative Assessment of Patient Experiences Related to Extended Pelvic Resection for Rectal Cancer［J］. J Surg Oncol，2006，93（2）：92-99.

附录1　全骶骨切除术后患者的健康相关生命质量调查问卷

说明：本调查用于研究全骶骨切除术后患者的健康相关生命质量。请您回答所有问题，并在选项上打"√"。如果您对答案不确定，请选择您认为最接近的答案。本调查承诺保护您的隐私，数据仅用于科学研究。谢谢您的配合。

一、您的一般情况

1. 您的文化程度

A. 不识字或识字很少

B. 小学毕业

C. 初中毕业

D. 高中、中专、中技、职高专业

E. 大学专科毕业

F. 大学本科毕业

G. 硕士研究生毕业及以上

2. 您的家庭人均月收入水平

A. ≤ 500 元

B. 501 ～ 1000 元

C. 1001 ～ 2000 元

D. 2001 ～ 3000 元

E. 3001 ～ 4000 元

F. 4001 ～ 6000 元

G. ≥ 6001 元

3. 您的职业是

A. 临时工、进城务工人员、无职业者

B. 体力劳动工人

C. 技术工人

D. 办公室一般工作人员

E. 一般管理人员与一般专业技术人员

F. 中层管理人员与中级专业技术人员

G. 高层管理人员与高级专业技术人员

二、健康相关生命质量调查量表（SF-36 v2 量表）

1. 总的来说，您认为您的健康状况

①棒极了　②很好　③好　④过得去　⑤糟糕

2. 与一年前相比，您如何评价现在的健康状况？

①比一年前好多了　②比一年前好一点　③和一年前差不多

④比一年前差一点　⑤比一年前差多了

3. 下列项目是您平常在一天中可能做的事情。您现在的健康限制您从事这些活动吗？如果是的话，程度如何？

3a. 高强度活动，如跑步、举重物、参与剧烈运动

①是，很受限　②是，稍受限　③不，完全不受限

3b. 中等度活动，如移动桌子，推动真空吸尘器（或拖地板）、打保龄球、打高尔夫球（或打太极拳）

①是，很受限　②是，稍受限　③不，完全不受限

3c. 举或搬运杂物

①是，很受限　②是，稍受限　③不，完全不受限

3d. 爬数层楼梯

①是，很受限　②是，稍受限　③不，完全不受限

3e. 爬一层楼梯

①是，很受限　②是，稍受限　③不，完全不受限

3f. 弯腰、屈膝

①是，很受限　②是，稍受限　③不，完全不受限

3g. 步行 1500 米以上
①是，很受限　②是，稍受限　③不，完全不受限

3h. 步行几个路口
①是，很受限　②是，稍受限　③不，完全不受限

3i. 步行一个路口
①是，很受限　②是，稍受限　③不，完全不受限

3j. 自己洗澡或穿衣
①是，很受限　②是，稍受限　③不，完全不受限

4. 在过去 4 周，您有多少时间因为生理健康原因，在工作或从事其他日常活动时有下列问题？

4a. 减少了工作或从事其他活动的时间
①所有时间　②大多数时间　③一些时间　④一点时间　⑤没有时间

4b. 减少了工作量或活动量
①所有时间　②大多数时间　③一些时间　④一点时间　⑤没有时间

4c. 从事工作或其他活动的种类受限
①所有时间　②大多数时间　③一些时间　④一点时间　⑤没有时间

4d. 从事工作或其他活动有困难（如费劲）
①所有时间　②大多数时间　③一些时间　④一点时间　⑤没有时间

5. 在过去 4 周，您有多少时间因为任何情感问题（如感到抑郁或焦虑），在工作或从事其他日常活动时有下列问题？

5a. 减少了工作或从事其他活动的时间
①所有时间　②大多数时间　③一些时间　④一点时间　⑤没有时间

5b. 减少了工作量或活动量
①所有时间　②大多数时间　③一些时间　④一点时间　⑤没有时间

5c. 从事工作或其他活动不像平常那么专心
①所有时间　②大多数时间　③一些时间　④一点时间　⑤没有时间

6. 在过去 4 周，您的生理健康或情感问题在何种程度上干扰了您与家人、朋友、邻居、团体的正常社会活动？
①完全没有　②轻度　③中度　④重度　⑤极度

7. 在过去 4 周，您经受了多少躯体疼痛？
①完全没有　②很轻微　③轻微　④中等　⑤严重　⑥很严重

8. 在过去 4 周，疼痛在多大程度上干扰了您的正常工作（包括户外工作和家务劳动）？
①完全没有　②一点点　③中度　④重度　⑤极度

9. 这些问题将问及您在过去 4 周的感觉和情感体验。对每一问题，请给出与您想法最接的一个答案。在过去 4 周，有多少时间：
9a. 您觉得干劲十足
①所有时间　②大多数时间　③一些时间　④一点时间　⑤没有时间

9b. 您非常紧张
①所有时间　②大多数时间　③一些时间　④一点时间　⑤没有时间

9c. 您感到情绪低落、沮丧，怎么也快乐不起来
①所有时间　②大多数时间　③一些时间　④一点时间　⑤没有时间

9d. 您觉得平静、安适
①所有时间　②大多数时间　③一些时间　④一点时间　⑤没有时间

9e. 您觉得精力旺盛
①所有时间　②大多数时间　③一些时间　④一点时间　⑤没有时间

9f. 您感到心灰意冷
①所有时间　②大多数时间　③一些时间　④一点时间　⑤没有时间

9g. 您觉得累极了

①所有时间　②大多数时间　③一些时间　④一点时间　⑤没有时间

9h. 您觉得快乐吗

①所有时间　②大多数时间　③一些时间　④一点时间　⑤没有时间

9i. 您觉得疲劳

①所有时间　②大多数时间　③一些时间　④一点时间　⑤没有时间

10. 在过去4周，有多少时间您的社会活动（如访问朋友、亲戚等）受您的生理健康或情感问题的影响？

①所有时间　②绝大多数时间　③一些时间　④一点时间　⑤没有时间

11. 下列每一种情形与您实际情况符合的程度如何？

11a. 和其他人相比，我似乎更容易生病

①全部符合　②大部分符合　③不知道　④大部分不符合　⑤全部不符合

11b. 我和我认识的人一样健康

①全部符合　②大部分符合　③不知道　④大部分不符合　⑤全部不符合

11c. 我预计我的健康状况将变得更差

①全部符合　②大部分符合　③不知道　④大部分不符合　⑤全部不符合

11d. 我的身体棒极了

①全部符合　②大部分符合　③不知道　④大部分不符合　⑤全部不符合

附录2　论文范例

Received: 28 July 2019 | Accepted: 31 October 2019

DOI: 10.1002/jso.25756

RESEARCH ARTICLE

 WILEY

Assessment of patient experiences following total sacrectomy for primary malignant sacral tumors: A qualitative study

Yifei Wang MD[1,2] | Weiming Liang MD[1,3] | Shan Qu MD[4] | Yidan Zhang MD[1] | Zhiye Du MD[1] | Tao Ji MD[1] | Huayi Qu MD[1] | Richard Gorlick MD[2] | Wei Guo MD[1]

[1]Department of Musculoskeletal Tumors, Peking University People's Hospital, Beijing, China

[2]Department of Pediatrics, MD Anderson Cancer Center, Houston, Texas

[3]Department of Orthopedics, The First Affiliated Hospital of Guangxi University of Science and Technology, Liuzhou, Guangxi, China

[4]Department of Psychology, Peking University People's Hospital, Beijing, China

Correspondence
Wei Guo, MD, PhD, Department of Musculoskeletal Tumors, Peking University People's Hospital, 100044 Beijing, China.
Email: bonetumor@163.com

Abstract

Background and Objectives: Few reports have investigated patient experiences following total en bloc sacrectomy. The aims of this study were to obtain a deeper understanding of patients' personal experiences, needs, and satisfaction with the treatment to reveal areas in which perioperative and long-term patient care can be improved.

Methods: A qualitative design was applied to examine patient experiences and supportive care needs. Patients treated between 2007 and 2017 were identified from our institutional database.

Results: A total of 28 survivors were interviewed (13 females, age 13-75 years). Eight themes were identified: the effect of surgery on patients' (a) daily lives, (b) social activities, (c) work or school activities, (d) and family lives; (e) acceptance of ostomy surgery; (f) need for guidance regarding long-term rehabilitation; (g) satisfaction with the medical services provided in the hospital; and (h) satisfaction with the treatment outcomes.

Conclusion: Total en bloc sacrectomy can yield satisfactory oncological outcomes; however, the procedure is a life-changing event for patients and their families. Physicians must provide long-term support and guidance after surgery to enable patients to fully understand and cope with the changes in their lives.

KEYWORDS
patient experience, qualitative study, total en bloc sacrectomy

1 | INTRODUCTION

Sacral tumors are rare. The most common primary sacral tumors include chordomas, chondrosarcomas, and giant cell tumors. To reduce the risk of local recurrence, en bloc tumor resection is necessary to ensure adequate surgical margins.[1-3] However, because of the complex anatomy of the sacrum and its surrounding nerves, blood vessels, and pelvic organs, it is difficult to obtain an adequate surgical margin.

Total en bloc sacrectomy is often required when the primary malignant tumor involves the high sacrum. This extremely challenging surgery can lead to major blood loss during surgery.[4-7] In addition, only a limited number of institutions can perform this surgery because multidisciplinary cooperation among general, urological, vascular, and plastic surgeons is often required. Our center is the largest sacral tumor treatment center in the country and has accumulated rich experience in sacral tumor resection. Although total en bloc sacrectomy is traditionally performed in stages using combined anterior and posterior approaches,[1-3,8,9] we have explored

---

Yifei Wang and Weiming Liang contributed equally to this study.

and reported one-stage total en bloc sacrectomy via a single posterior approach to reduce operative time, blood loss, and surgical complications.[4-7,10-12]

However, total en bloc sacrectomy can impair bladder and bowel function, sexual function, and lower limb function due to nerve sacrifice (S1 and below) during surgery, thereby seriously affecting ambulation and daily living and presenting challenges for maintenance of healthy psychological and social functioning. Therefore, this patient population substantially differs from those with nonsacral bone tumors and those undergoing lower sacral tumor resection.

Quality of life scales, one type of tool for evaluating the quality of life of patients, often fail to describe all patient experiences. However, a qualitative approach can provide an in-depth look at the personal experiences of patients and help us to assess the effect of a disease on their personal lives and emotions. Previous studies have used qualitative methods to analyze patients with bone tumors[13-17] and the special challenges that they face. The current study is the first to use qualitative analysis to study the personal experiences and emotions of patients receiving total en bloc sacrectomy.

2 | MATERIALS AND METHODS

By reviewing electronic medical records, we followed up with patients who underwent total en bloc sacrectomy at our hospital between September 2007 and September 2017; patients without evidence of tumor recurrence who were willing to participate in this study were included. We obtained the following patient information from their electronic medical records: demographic data, diagnosis data, operation time, the presence of adjuvant chemotherapy, and length of hospital stay. The ethics committee of our hospital approved this study.

The interview questions were formulated by two orthopedic surgeons and a psychologist (WL, YW, and SQ) and reviewed by multiple experts (WG, TJ, and HQ) in the field. We referred to studies involving qualitative analysis methods in related fields.[15,16] The interview guide included the following topics: what are the functional psychosocial consequences of the disease and treatment; whether the disease and the treatment had changed the patients' lives; and if they are satisfied with the treatment outcome. We also focused on how the bowel and bladder impairment affects their quality of life and their acceptance of ostomy surgery.

Two orthopedic surgeons (WL and YW) conducted the semi-structured open-ended interviews with the patients over the phone under the supervision of an expert in qualitative analysis (SQ). The interview time on average was 46 minutes (range 33-65 minutes). The phone interviews were audio-recorded. After the interview, the recordings were reviewed several times. Together, all three researchers (YW, WL, and SQ) created a single codebook with agreement on the definitions of each code. Then, the researchers

coded the statements of each patient independently. Opinions shared by multiple patients were identified.

SPSS 22 (IBM, Armonk) was used for data analysis. The Kaplan-Meier method was used to analyze the overall and event-free survival rates. The kappa statistic was used to assess the intercoder agreement.[18,19] Kappa values from 0.40 to 0.75 were considered to indicate "intermediate to good" agreement, and values above 0.75 were considered to indicate "excellent" agreement.[20]

3 | RESULTS

On the basis of medical records search, 41 patients underwent total en bloc sacrectomy between September 2007 and September 2017 at our hospital and completed a follow-up assessment. Eight patients died (tumor recurrence and/or metastasis), 5 survived with tumor recurrence, and 28 patients survived without tumor recurrence and were willing to participate in the qualitative study. The estimated 5-year overall survival rate of all 41 patients was 83.3%, whereas the 5-year event-free survival rate was 68.1% (Figures 1 and 2). The average operative time of the 28 patients was 6.3 ± 2.5 hours, and the average intraoperative blood loss was 2771.3 ± 1619.5 mL. Table 1 provides basic patient information.

The kappa value for the intercoder agreement was calculated as 0.93, which is considered the excellent agreement.[20] After completion of the 28 patient interviews, eight themes were identified: the effect of surgery on patients' (a) daily lives, (b) social activities, (c) work or school activities, (d) and family lives; (e) acceptance of ostomy surgery; (f) need for guidance regarding long-term rehabilitation; (g) satisfaction with the medical services provided in the hospital; and (h) satisfaction with the treatment outcomes (Table 2).

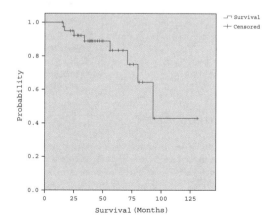

FIGURE 1 The overall 1-year and 5-year survival curves of 41 patients who received total en bloc sacrectomy (100% and 83.3%, respectively) [Color figure can be viewed at wileyonlinelibrary.com]

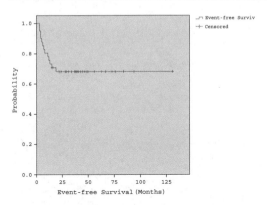

FIGURE 2 The overall event-free 1-year and 5-year survival curves of 41 patients who received total en bloc sacrectomy (75.6% and 68.1%, respectively) [Color figure can be viewed at wileyonlinelibrary.com]

3.1 | Effect on daily life

Seventeen patients stated that they were unable to perform routine self-care without the help of others, primarily because of the weakening of their lower limbs, especially the ankle joint. Because of pain or restricted back movements, they were unable to independently raise and dress themselves. Fourteen patients reported that they could not bathe, defecate, or urinate without help.

Eleven patients indicated that they did not need help in their daily lives. These patients recovered well after surgery and adapted to their current lives.

TABLE 1 Patient demographic and clinical characteristics

Characteristics	Number of patients
Sex	
Male	15
Female	13
Age (range), y	47 (13-75)
Pathological type	
Chordoma	17
Chondrosarcoma	6
Osteosarcoma	3
Ewing sarcoma	2
Colostomy	
Yes	1
No	27
Ureterostomy	
Yes	1
No	27
Adjuvant chemotherapy	
Yes	5
No	23
Average length of hospital stay, d	36 (18-75)
Average follow-up period, mo	48 (15-131)

3.2 | Social activity

A total of 23 patients indicated that their social activities were significantly reduced after surgery. Most patients said that lower limb impairment limited their social activity. Eight patients indicated that fatigue also reduced their social activity, and five indicated that they were reluctant to participate in social activities because of concerns regarding urinary incontinence.

Only five patients indicated that their social activities were normal. Four patients indicated that they recovered well after surgery and were satisfied with their lower limb function for their basic needs. In addition, although one patient was unable to travel, her relatives and friends often came to visit her, making her feel as though her social activities were not significantly reduced.

3.3 | School or work

A total of 23 patients said that they could not return to school or work. Four patients have enrolled students, and they did not return to school after receiving treatment. Nineteen patients did not return to work after the treatment. Some patients reached retirement age and, therefore, did not continue to work. Others indicated that they were unable to perform their duties due to limited mobility, fatigue, and pain.

Five patients returned to their jobs (two business managers, one physician, one government employee, and one cashier). These positions do not require much physical strength.

3.4 | Family life

A total of 24 patients indicated that tumor treatment significantly affected their families. Most of the patients said that they were unable to live without the help of their family members, who provided time and effort.

Only four patients believed that their tumor treatment had a little effect on their families. They did not deny the effect that the surgery had, during and after, on the family. However, they recovered well, and their family lives were resuming normalcy. The effects of the tumor and treatment on their family lives were resolved.

3.5 | Acceptance of ostomy surgery

A total of 25 patients indicated that they were unwilling to undergo ostomy surgery. Some patients believed that their current bowel and bladder function was acceptable, and no further treatment was needed. Some patients believed that ostomy bags would seriously affect their appearance and were psychologically unacceptable.

Only three patients considered ostomy surgery to be acceptable. Patient 5 had a colostomy because of a bowel injury experienced during surgery and said that he had adapted to his current state. Because of the pain of an indwelling urethral catheter, patient 9

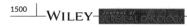

高位骶骨肿瘤外科治疗结局

TABLE 2 Patient statements for each topic

Topic	Patient statements	
1. Daily life		
Require help	"I can't live without my mom. I need my mom to help with bathing and urinating. I urinate frequently. My mom is almost always with me. I can't walk without a supportive device. I cannot reach my feet, wear pants or socks, or cut my toenails. I need my spouse's help for getting up."—patient 2	17 patients made similar statements
Complete ability of self-care	"I can take care of myself, walk, and carry items without help."—patient 4	11 patients made similar statements
2. Social activities		
Significant decrease	"My physical strength after surgery is not as good as before. I always feel tired. Even if a friend asks me to hang out, I rarely go."—patient 27 "I rarely hang out with friends because of serious urinary incontinence. I feel embarrassed when I have accidents."—patient 28	23 patients made similar statements
No substantial changes	"I often drive by myself, travel with friends, sing with friends, and go to temple to worship Buddha."—patient 12 "I often have friends and family come see me, chat with me, play mahjong, or sing. They make me feel that my family always supports me."—patient 24	5 patients made similar statements
3. School or work		
Inability to go to school or work	"I dropped out of school when I got sick and have not been able to go back since the surgery because I can't move, and I need my family to take care of me. I can't take care of myself at school. I really envy the students who are able to go to school daily."—patient 2 "I was a mechanic in a car shop. After surgery, I resigned because I couldn't do repairs from the positions that are required to work on cars."—patient 23	23 patients made similar statements
Ability to work	"I recovered very well. I quickly returned to my original job. The surgery didn't have much effect on my work because my boss no longer expected me to do high-intensity manual labor."—patient 12	5 patients made similar statements
4. Family life		
Substantial changes	"My daughter arranged for me to live in a nursing home. If she were to take care of me, then she would have no way to work."—patient 8 "My husband thinks that I am a burden, and he doesn't want to take care of me anymore."—patient 14 "My mom quit her job to take care of me."—patient 2	24 patients made similar statements
No substantial changes	"I am working routinely now. The surgery changed little in my family. My family life is almost the same as before. I occasionally feel sick, but I can handle it myself. I don't need special care from my family."—patient 12	4 patients made similar statements
5. Acceptance of ostomy surgery		
Unwilling to accept	"I have cosmetic concerns because I would have incision scars on my stomach. I am still young. I want to date someone and get married, and I would not accept this kind of surgery."—patient 2 "Occasionally, I need to use a diaper due to urinary incontinence. The surgery would have little effect on my life."—patient 12	25 patients made similar statements
Willing to accept	"I can clean the ostomy bag myself to eliminate unpleasant odors."—patient 5 "After the operation, I could not urinate without a urinary catheter. It was too painful. Later, I underwent a ureterostomy at a hospital nearby. Now, I feel very good."—patient 9 "I have accidents every day. If ostomy surgery can solve urinary incontinence, then I would accept it."—patient 14	3 patients made similar statements
6. Need for long-term rehabilitation guidance		
Need	"It has been more than 4 y since the surgery. I was cured of the tumor, but I have no idea what to pay attention to when I turn over or sit down. I don't know if I'm doing it right."—patient 11 "I don't know to what degree I can recover, and I don't know if my current situation is normal."—patient 20	All patients made similar statements

(Continues)

Journal of SURGICAL ONCOLOGY **-WILEY** | 1501

TABLE 2 (Continued)

Topic	Patient statements	
7. Satisfaction with medical services		
Satisfied	"The physicians and nurses are very good and responsible. I was very desperate when I was in the hospital. I kept crying for several days. My mom couldn't help me with this. Finally, the nurse came to comfort me and made me feel better."—patient 2	27 patients made similar statements
	"The physician was highly skilled and treated patients respectfully. The nurse worked like an artist to change my wound dressing."—patient 25	
Dissatisfied	"The physician damaged my bowel and made my life very miserable. I stayed in the hospital for a long time and spent a lot of money."—patient 5	1 patient
8. Satisfaction with treatment outcomes		
Satisfied	"I understand that I had a malignant tumor, and I am satisfied with the treatment outcome because I'm alive now, and I can walk. You saved my life, and I am very grateful to you."—patient 7	23 patients made similar statements
Dissatisfied	"Since the operation, my legs hurt and lack feeling, and the pain medicine doesn't work; I'm suffering."—patient 6	5 patients made similar statements
	"I'm not able to walk, and urinary incontinence has seriously affected my life."—patient 28	

underwent a ureterostomy 6 months after surgery. Patient 14 reported that urinary incontinence seriously affected her life; therefore, she was willing to undergo ureterostomy to improve her quality of life.

3.6 | Need for long-term rehabilitation guidance

All 28 patients who participated in the study expressed that more guidance concerning long-term rehabilitation was needed. In general, before performing the surgery, our multidisciplinary team repeatedly explained the benefits of surgery, the possible risks, the possible postoperative outcomes, and the recovery experience. However, most patients expressed that they needed more information during the follow-up period about the extent of their final functional rehabilitation (eg, lower limb, bowel, and bladder function).

3.7 | Satisfaction with medical services

Due to the prolonged hospital stay following total en bloc sacrectomy (average >1 month), our healthcare team provided relevant knowledge to the patients before the operation and explained the difficulties that they might encounter during the treatment process as well as the help and guidance that could be provided to them. We guided the patients on how to perform limb function training after surgery, and before patient discharge, we assisted and guided patients and their families on how to help the patient turn over and urinate. Therefore, the patients and our medical team had close interactions during hospitalization. According to the interview results, 27 patients evaluated the medical team as satisfactory.

Only one patient expressed dissatisfaction with medical services. Patient 5 was angry that he experienced bowel injury during surgery.

3.8 | Satisfaction with treatment outcomes

A total of 23 patients were satisfied with the treatment outcome. Although some patients showed poor postoperative functional recovery, they all believed that surgery helped cure the tumor and saved their lives, and they expressed their gratitude to us.

Five patients expressed dissatisfaction with the treatment outcome. Four complained of poor lower limb function recovery after surgery, two complained of poor bowel function recovery, and two were unable to accept the treatment outcome because of intractable pain.

4 | DISCUSSION

The incidence of primary malignant tumors invading the higher sacrum is low, and total en bloc sacrectomy is extremely challenging. Therefore, reports in the literature regarding the experience of patients undergoing total en bloc sacrectomy are rare, and most are small case series with fewer than 10 patients.[1,3,8,9,21-24] Asavamong-kolkul and Waikakul[25] reported 12 sacral chordoma patients who underwent total sacrectomy via a posterior approach. All patients had bowel and bladder dysfunction postoperatively.[25] van Wulfften Palthe et al[26] reported 10 patients who received en bloc sacrectomy with the L5 nerve root spared. They investigated the postoperative outcomes using the National Institutes of Health Patient Reported Measurement Information System and concluded that a preoperative discussion should occur with these patients about the potential effects on physical and mental functions.[26] After a thorough literature review, we believe the sample size of the current study is

1502 | WILEY—Journal of SURGICAL ONCOLOGY

the largest to date, which might allow us to evaluate the oncological prognosis of total en bloc sacrectomy and the effect of this procedure on patient experiences. In this study, 41 patients underwent total en bloc sacrectomy at our hospital and completed a follow-up assessment. Eight patients died of tumor recurrence and/or metastasis, and five patients survived with tumor recurrence. The 5-year overall survival rate of patients was 83.3%, which is acceptable compared with values reported in previous studies.[1,3,8,9,21-24,27,28]

This study was the first to employ a qualitative analysis to study patients who underwent total en bloc sacrectomy and explore the long-term effects of this surgery on the physiological, psychological, and social functions of patients from their perspective. This feature is unique to this study. Understanding patient experience will help us to meaningfully change the medical services provided, thereby improving patient recovery and postoperative quality of life. The topics that we identified after the interviews included the effect of surgery on the patients' (a) daily lives, (b) social activities, (c) work or school, (d) family life; (e) acceptance of ostomy surgery; (f) need for guidance regarding long-term rehabilitation; (g) satisfaction with the medical service of the hospital; and (h) satisfaction with the treatment outcomes.

In the current study, more than half of the patients said that they were unable to perform routine self-care and could not live without the help of others. The primary causes of this problem were lower limb impairment, fatigue, and restricted lower back movement. Because of these problems, the patients were at high risk of falling when alone or were unable to complete specific activities (eg, bathing and putting on shoes). Bowel and bladder impairment was also underlying causes of these problems. Additionally, some patients had severe constipation and needed assistance with defecation (ie, an enema) that required another person.

The effect on the family is also a topic that cannot be ignored. Under the influence of traditional Confucianism, the culture of China and some other Asian countries emphasizes the moral obligation that each family member has to care for relatives who are patients. Unwillingness to care creates a sense of moral failure.[29,30] This consequence might not exist in Western culture, which tends to consider care as the patient's responsibility.[31] In this study, most families paid a high price in terms of both money and time when caring for patients. Tumor treatment is often costly, and poor families often sacrifice their earnings to ensure that family members with cancer are treated; thus, they are burdened with a heavy debt. Many individuals sacrifice their jobs to take care of sick family members. However, the patients themselves often feel guilt about bothering their families and sometimes attempt to cope with problems themselves, even when they suffer greatly from the disease.[30] An elderly female patient in this study said that she would not undergo treatment if she had the opportunity to choose again. She would have rather used her limited family savings for future generations' education and improve the quality of life of her family. This finding suggests that patients' emotions and treatment selections are influenced by their cultural backgrounds. Thus, physicians should consider this factor when making medical suggestions. As mentioned above, the treatment of sacral tumors also substantially affects

family members with regard to money, time, and mood. When coupled with moral pressure in a traditional culture, the situation became unbearable for some of the families, triggering familial discord. For example, the husband of one young female patient was unwilling to continue to care for the patient and filed for divorce.

This study showed that after total en bloc sacrectomy, the social activity of most patients was significantly reduced. Patients' impaired ability to walk made it difficult for them to participate in entertainment and sports with their friends. In addition, an abnormal gait and the odor caused by bladder and bowel incontinence also led to feelings of inferiority, thereby lowering patients' interest in participating in social activities. Other studies have reported similar observations.[13,16] In the current study, the few patients without significant social activity limitations had a common feature: better recovery of lower limb function.

Previous studies have reported that patients with disabilities are disadvantaged in the job market.[13,14,16] The results of the current study are consistent with previous results, showing that only five patients returned to work after the treatment. Most of the patients who did not return to work were blue-collar employees. The five patients who returned to work had jobs that did not require much physical strength. Therefore, they were still able to meet their job requirements, even though they had mild lower limb impairment. The four patients in this study who were students were unable to return to school. Regardless of whether the patients were unemployed or dropped out of school, the treatments created barriers to their future careers and reduced their feelings of self-worth.

Thus so far, no consensus has been developed regarding whether total en bloc sacrectomy should be performed concurrently with a colostomy. Although an ostomy can address bowel and bladder incontinence, ostomy surgeries also cause problems, such as skin irritation and unpleasant odor, and affect patient appearance, thereby reducing quality of life and increasing anxiety and/or depression.[32] Studies have shown that a unique appearance can lead to negative reactions and discrimination as well as social problems that affect patients' self-esteem. Therefore, patients often resist changes that modify their body image.[17,33] Most patients in this study were reluctant to undergo ostomy surgery. Although they had abnormal bowel and bladder function, most were able to adapt to their current state and did not report that their current bowel/bladder dysfunction significantly affected their quality of life. Their current situation was not sufficiently negative to merit undergoing ostomy surgery. Given that studies have reported that ostomy surgery can increase infection rates and prolong hospital stays[34] and that most patients are able to accept the current state of their bowel and bladder functions without experiencing a significant effect on their quality of life, we tend not to perform concurrent ostomy surgery.

All patients in this study expressed a desire to receive more guidance regarding postoperative rehabilitation, as was reported in another qualitative study.[15] Although we fully explained to the patients the possible risks of surgery and the specific requirements for postoperative rehabilitation, they likely paid more attention to whether the tumor could be cured, whether they would still be able to walk, and the possible costs of treatment; as a result, they poorly understood the long-term effects of chronic pain and lower limb weakness, as well as those of bowel and bladder dysfunctions, on their personal and family lives. They might have forgotten relevant information during the long postoperative rehabilitation process because a considerable amount of complex information is presented to them. In addition, some patients chose to undergo follow-up assessments at a nearby hospital. However, the physicians at that hospital often did not have experience with total en bloc sacrectomy; therefore, they might not have provided enough information. Thus, we developed a patient-knowledge handbook and provided it to patients before surgery so that they could read it at any time.

Most of the patients in this study expressed satisfaction with the medical services that we provided. Many patients thought that the nurses provided excellent physical and psychological rehabilitation support during their hospital stay. This finding indicates that both the physicians and the trained nursing team/rehabilitation therapists helped the patients adjust to their new psychological state after total en bloc sacrectomy by providing emotional support. We believe that this care improved the patient experience. Most patients expressed satisfaction with the treatment outcome. Five patients were dissatisfied with the treatment outcome due to pain or dysfunction. On the basis of the results of this study, we should fully inform patients of the possibility of chronic pain and related dysfunction and provide functional training methods after total en bloc sacrectomy. Moreover, during the long-term follow-up period, we should provide appropriate guidance and psychological support. This study provides an important basis to optimize long-term treatment schemes for patients undergoing total en bloc sacrectomy. In addition to the aforementioned patient-knowledge handbook, the measures that have been implemented include the following. Each patient was assigned to a group of providers who had experience with total en bloc sacrectomy, including a physician, a nurse, and a rehabilitation therapist, who could be contacted by the patient at any time. In addition to the regular follow-up assessment, long-term support and professional guidance were provided to meet the specific needs of patients undergoing total en bloc sacrectomy. Furthermore, the treatment team included a psychologist (SQ) at our hospital who provided psychological counseling services to patients when necessary. The effectiveness of these measures in improving the quality of life and emotions of patients must be further evaluated.

We acknowledge that this study has limitations. First, although this case series is the largest reported to date to investigate the effect of total en bloc sacrectomy, only 28 patients were included in this qualitative study. The small sample size might lead to certain biases. For example, concurrent ostomy should be further studied. In addition, because of the nature of retrospective research, continuous information was lacking, and changes in the function, mental state, and emotional recovery of the patients after surgery were not analyzed over time.

5 | CONCLUSION

This study is the first to conduct a qualitative analysis with the aim of deeply understanding the significant effect of total en bloc

sacrectomy on patient quality of life and emotional experience from their perspective. Total en bloc sacrectomy provides an acceptable oncological prognosis; however, patients pay a substantial price regarding their daily lives, social activities, family lives, and school or job opportunities. In addition, a patient's cultural background might affect their emotional experience and treatment decisions. Orthopedic oncologists should address these factors and work with the care team, rehabilitation team, and psychologists to communicate with patients and understand the difficulties and challenges that these patients might face. Ultimately, long-term treatment schemes should be developed for patients undergoing total en bloc sacrectomy to provide long-term support and guidance after surgery.

ORCID

Wei Guo http://orcid.org/0000-0002-7355-910X

REFERENCES

1. Doita M, Harada T, Iguchi T, et al. Total sacrectomy and reconstruction for sacral tumors. *Spine (Phila Pa 1976)*. 2003;28:E296-E301.
2. Fourney DR, Rhines LD, Hentschel SJ, et al. En bloc resection of primary sacral tumors: classification of surgical approaches and outcome. *J Neurosurg Spine*. 2005;3:111-122.
3. Tomita K, Tsuchiya H. Total sacrectomy and reconstruction for huge sacral tumors. *Spine (Phila Pa 1976)*. 1990;15:1223-1227.
4. Li D, Guo W, Tang X, et al. Surgical classification of different types of en bloc resection for primary malignant sacral tumors. *Eur Spine J*. 2011;20:2275-2281.
5. Guo W, Tang X, Zang J, Ji T. One-stage total en bloc sacrectomy: a novel technique and report of 9 cases. *Spine (Phila Pa 1976)*. 2013;38:E626-E631.
6. Zang J, Guo W, Yang R, Tang X, Li D. Is total en bloc sacrectomy using a posterior-only approach feasible and safe for patients with malignant sacral tumors? *J Neurosurg Spine*. 2015;22:563-570.
7. Wang Y, Guo W, Shen D, et al. Surgical treatment of primary osteosarcoma of the sacrum: a case series of 26 patients. *Spine (Phila Pa 1976)*. 2017;42:1207-1213.
8. Wuisman P, Lieshout O, Sugihara S, van Dijk M. Total sacrectomy and reconstruction: oncologic and functional outcome. *Clin Orthop Relat Res*. 2000;381:192-203.
9. Shikata J, Yamamuro T, Kotoura Y, Mikawa Y, Iida H, Maetani S. Total sacrectomy and reconstruction for primary tumors. Report of two cases. *J Bone Joint Surg Am*. 1988;70:122-125.
10. Ji T, Guo W, Yang R, Tang X, Wang Y, Huang L. What are the conditional survival and functional outcomes after surgical treatment of 115 patients with sacral chordoma? *Clin Orthop Relat Res*. 2017;475:620-630.
11. Wang Y, Wei R, Ji T, Chen Z, Guo W. Surgical treatment of primary solitary fibrous tumors involving the pelvic ring. *PLoS One*. 2018;13. e0207581.
12. Ji T, Yang Y, Wang Y, Sun K, Guo W. Combining of serial embolization and denosumab for large sacropelvic giant cell tumor: case report of 3 cases. *Medicine*. 2017;96. e7799.
13. Earle EA, Eiser C, Grimer R. 'He never liked sport anyway'—mother's views of young people coping with a bone tumour in the lower limb. *Sarcoma*. 2005;9:7-13.
14. Parsons JA, Eakin JM, Bell RS, Franche RL, Davis AM. "So, are you back to work yet?" Re-conceptualizing 'work' and 'return to work' in the context of primary bone cancer. *Soc Sci Med*. 2008;67:1826-1836.

15. Davidge KM, Eskicioglu C, Lipa J, Ferguson P, Swallow CJ, Wright FC. Qualitative assessment of patient experiences following sacrectomy. *J Surg Oncol.* 2010;101:447-450.

16. Fauske L, Bruland OS, Grov EK, Bondevik H. Cured of primary bone cancer, but at what cost: a qualitative study of functional impairment and lost opportunities. *Sarcoma.* 2015;2015. 484196.

17. Fauske L, Lorem G, Grov EK, Bondevik H. Changes in the body image of bone sarcoma survivors following surgical treatment—a qualitative study. *J Surg Oncol.* 2016;113:229-234.

18. Randolph JJ Online Kappa Calculator [Computer Software]. 2008; http://justus.randolph.name/kappa

19. Warrens MJ. Inequalities between multi-rater kappas. *Adv Data Anal Classif.* 2010;4:271-286.

20. Grove WA. Statistical-methods for rates and proportions, 2nd Edition - Fleiss, Jl. *Am J Psychiatry.* 1981;138:1644-1645.

21. Hulen CA, Temple HT, Fox WP, Sama AA, Green BA, Eismont FJ. Oncologic and functional outcome following sacrectomy for sacral chordoma. *J Bone Joint Surg Am.* 2006;88:1532-1539.

22. Clarke MJ, Dasenbrock H, Bydon A, et al. Posterior-only approach for en bloc sacrectomy: clinical outcomes in 36 consecutive patients. *Neurosurgery.* 2012;71:357-364.

23. Phukan R, Herzog T, Boland PJ, et al. How does the level of sacral resection for primary malignant bone tumors affect physical and mental health, pain, mobility, incontinence, and sexual function? *Clin Orthop Relat Res.* 2016;474:687-696.

24. Kiatisevi P, Piyaskulkaew C, Kunakornsawat S, Sukunthanak B. What are the functional outcomes after total sacrectomy without spinopelvic reconstruction? *Clin Orthop Relat Res.* 2017;475: 643-655.

25. Asavamongkolkul A, Waikakul S. Wide resection of sacral chordoma via a posterior approach. *Int Orthop.* 2012;36:607-612.

26. van Wulfften Palthe OD, Houdek MT, Rose PS, et al. How does the level of nerve root resection in en bloc sacrectomy influence patient-reported outcomes? *Clin Orthop Relat Res.* 2017;475: 607-616.

27. Miles WK, Chang DW, Kroll SS, et al. Reconstruction of large sacral defects following total sacrectomy. *Plast Reconstr Surg.* 2000;105: 2387-2394.

28. Dickey ID, Hugate RR Jr, Fuchs B, Yaszemski MJ, Sim FH. Reconstruction after total sacrectomy: early experience with a new surgical technique. *Clin Orthop Relat Res.* 2005;438:42-50.

29. Wong TK, Pang SM. Holism and caring: nursing in the Chinese health care culture. *Holist Nurs Pract.* 2000;15:12-21.

30. Tao H, Songwathana P, Isaramalai SA, Wang Q. Taking good care of myself: a qualitative study on self-care behavior among Chinese persons with a permanent colostomy. *Nurs Health Sci.* 2014;16:483-489.

31. Richard AA, Shea K. Delineation of self-care and associated concepts. *J Nurs Scholarship.* 2011;43:255-264.

32. Dabirian A, Yaghmaei F, Rassouli M, Tafreshi MZ. Quality of life in ostomy patients: a qualitative study. *Patient Prefer Adherence.* 2010;5:1-5.

33. Silva NM, Santos MAD, Rosado SR, Galvão CM, Sonobe HM. Psychological aspects of patients with intestinal stoma: integrative review. *Rev Lat Am Enfermagem.* 2017;25. e2950.

34. Vartanian ED, Lynn JV, Perrault DP, et al. Risk factors associated with reconstructive complications following sacrectomy. *Plast Reconstr Surg Glob Open.* 2018;6. e2002.

SUPPORTING INFORMATION

Additional supporting information may be found online in the Supporting Information section.

How to cite this article: Wang Y, Liang W, Qu S, et al. Assessment of patient experiences following total sacrectomy for primary malignant sacral tumors: A qualitative study. *J Surg Oncol.* 2019;120:1497–1504. https://doi.org/10.1002/jso.25756

Yu *et al.*
Journal of Orthopaedic Surgery and Research　(2023) 18:100
https://doi.org/10.1186/s13018-023-03590-2

Journal of Orthopaedic
Surgery and Research

SYSTEMATIC REVIEW　　　　　　　　　　　　　　　　　　**Open Access**

Efficacy and safety of anti-interleukin-1 therapeutics in the treatment of knee osteoarthritis: a systematic review and meta-analysis of randomized controlled trials

Lizhi Yu, Raoshan Luo, Gang Qin, Qinyan Zhang and Weiming Liang[*]

Abstract

Objective We aimed to evaluate the efficacy and safety of anti-interleukin-1 therapeutics, including IL-1 antibodies, interleukin-1 receptor antagonists (IL-1 Ras) and IL-1 inhibitors, for knee osteoarthritis (KOA) treatment.

Methods Databases (Medline, Embase, Web of Science and CENTRAL) and ClinicalTrials.gov were systematically searched for randomized controlled trials (RCTs) of anti-interleukin-1 therapeutics from inception to August 31, 2022. The outcomes were the mean change in pain and function scores and the risk of adverse effects (AEs).

Results In the 12 studies included, anti-interleukin-1 therapeutics were superior to placebo in terms of pain relief (standardized mean difference [SMD] $= -0.38$, 95% confidence interval [CI] $= -1.82$ to -0.40, $p < 0.001$, $I^2 = 77\%$) and functional improvement (SMD $= -1.11$, 95% CI $= -1.82$ to -0.40, $p = 0.002$, $I^2 = 96\%$). The incidence of any AE (risk ratio [RR] $= 1.02$, 95% CI $= 0.88–1.18$, $p < 0.001$, $I2 = 76\%$) was higher following treatment with anti-interleukin-1 therapeutics than placebo, while no significant difference was found in the incidence of serious AEs (SAEs) or discontinuations due to AEs. Subgroup analyses showed that IL-1 antibodies and the IL-1 inhibitor provided pain relief (IL-1 antibodies: SMD $= -0.61$, 95% CI $= -0.92$ to -0.31, $p < 0.001$; IL-1 inhibitor: SMD $= -0.39$, 95% CI $= -0.72$ to -0.06, $p = 0.02$, $I2 = 74.0\%$) and functional improvement (IL-1 antibodies: SMD $= -1.75$, 95% CI $= -2.10$ to -1.40, $p < 0.001$; IL-1 inhibitor: SMD $= -0.28$, 95% CI $= -0.83$ to 0.27, $p = 0.31$, $I^2 = 88\%$) superior to those of placebo, whereas IL-1 Ras did not. However, the IL-1 inhibitor increased the incidence of any AE (RR $= 1.35$, 95% CI $= 0.92–1.98$, $p < 0.001$, $I^2 = 85\%$) but not the risk of SAEs or discontinuations due to AEs. IL-1 antibodies and IL-1 Ras showed no difference in safety compared with placebo.

Conclusions Anti-interleukin-1 therapeutics could relieve OA-related pain and improve function, but is probably associated with an increased risk of adverse events. Specially, IL-1 antibodies and an IL-1 inhibitor could relieve OA-related pain and improve function, whereas IL-1 Ras could not. IL-1 antibodies and IL-1 Ras were relatively safe options, but IL-1 inhibitors were associated with safety concerns.

*Correspondence:
Weiming Liang
liangwm22@icloud.com
Full list of author information is available at the end of the article

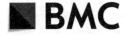

Yu et al. Journal of Orthopaedic Surgery and Research   (2023) 18:100

Keywords Anti-interleukin-1 therapeutics, Meta-analysis, IL-1 antibodies, Interleukin-1 receptor antagonist, IL-1 inhibitors

Introduction

Osteoarthritis (OA) is a whole-joint disease in which all of the components of the joint are affected [1]. OA is the most common joint disease, with more than 240 million people suffering varying degrees of OA worldwide, and the knee joint (knee OA, KOA) is the most commonly affected joint [2, 3]. The main clinical symptoms of KOA are pain, stiffness, and limited mobility, which are associated with the inflammation of the knee joint and greatly affects the patient's quality of life [4–6]. Patients with end-stage KOA can be well treated with knee replacement [7], but the same treatment is unacceptable for early-stage KOA or young and middle-aged KOA patients. Thus, conservative nonsurgical interventions are proposed to treat painful joints [8–10]. At present, nonsurgical interventions are mainly used to relieve clinical symptoms, improve joint function, and slow down the degeneration of intra-articular structures to avoid or delay joint replacement surgery [11–15]. Nonsurgical treatment options for KOA include a wide variety of drugs, including non-steroidal anti-inflammatory drugs (NSAIDs), opioids, steroids, and hyaluronic acid (HA), as well as exercise therapy and weight loss, but the results are not satisfactory [13, 16–23]. Moreover, NSAIDs and opioids are poorly tolerated in many patients, and the safety profile of long-term therapy with NSAIDs or opioids is concerning [17, 18, 24, 25]. Therefore, a new KOA treatment direction is urgently needed.

With the further study of the pathological mechanism of OA, an increasing number of new targets have been discovered and have become the focus of recent pharmaprojects. Inflammatory cytokines, such as interleukin (IL), tumour necrosis factor (TNF), and nerve growth factor (NGF), which are the key mediators that promote the pathophysiology of KOA, cannot be ignored in the occurrence of OA. It has been shown that inflammatory cytokines act as a signals that mimic chondrodegradation enzymes from chondrocytes [26]. IL-1 β and tumour necrosis factor-α (TNF-α) are the key cytokines in the cartilage catabolic process [27–31]. Among the many ILs, IL-1α, IL-1β, and other IL-1 family members are the most highly profiled and have all been shown to be present in the synovial fluid and subchondral bone of OA patients [32–34]. IL-1β is involved in the pathogenesis of cartilage loss and destructive OA [34–36]. With the deepening of basic research, it has become an established fact that IL-1 triggers KOA;

therefore, whether anti-IL-1 therapy could treat KOA has aroused great interest from researchers [37, 38].

The current anti-IL-1 therapeutics found in the available literature for KOA mainly consist of the following three types: IL-1 antibodies, IL-1 Ras, and IL-1 inhibitors [39–45]. The literature included in the current published meta-analysis is not comprehensive, as some drugs are missing or the latest research results are missing as they were not available at the time of publication, so the inconsistent efficacy and safety of anti-IL-1 therapeutics in KOA reported in the literature cannot comprehensively explain the advantages and disadvantages of anti-IL-1 therapeutics [46–48]. Therefore, the correct clinical treatment strategy may not be made by solely relying on the results of existing studies and there is a need to update the data on the efficacy and safety of anti-IL-1 therapeutics.

The purpose of this meta-analysis was to evaluate the efficacy and safety of anti-IL-1 therapeutics for KOA treatment. Pain and function scores as well as adverse events were evaluated in a meta-analysis of RCTs. We hypothesized that anti-IL-1 therapeutics would be more efficacious in terms of pain relief and functional improvement in the treatment of patients with KOA than control treatment, and anti-IL-1 therapeutics were relatively safe options.

Methods

The present study was completed according to the Cochrane guidelines for issues related to the methodology of systematic reviews [49].

Search strategy

We conducted a systematic literature search in Medline (1946 to August 31, 2022), Embase (1974 to August 31, 2022), Web of Science (1966 to August 31, 2022), and CENTRAL(1995 to August 31, 2022) to identify relevant studies. The search strategy was as follows: (((((((("lutikizumab" [Supplementary Concept]) OR (((ABT-981) OR (an anti-interleukin-1alpha and anti-interleukin-1beta dual variable domain immunoglobulin)) OR ("lutikizumab" [Supplementary Concept])))) OR ("Interleukin 1 Receptor Antagonist Protein"[Mesh])) OR ((((((((((((IL1 Febrile Inhibitor) OR (Febrile Inhibitor, IL1)) OR (IL-1Ra)) OR (Urine-Derived IL1 Inhibitor)) OR (IL1 Inhibitor, Urine-Derived)) OR (Urine Derived IL1 Inhibitor)) OR (IL-1 Inhibitor, Urine))

Yu *et al. Journal of Orthopaedic Surgery and Research*　(2023) 18:100　　　　

OR (IL 1 Inhibitor, Urine)) OR (Urine IL-1 Inhibitor)) OR (Interleukin 1 Inhibitor, Urine)) OR (Antril)) OR (Kineret)) OR (Anakinra)))) OR (diacerein)) OR ("canakinumab" [Supplementary Concept])) AND (((((((((((Osteoarthritides) OR (Osteoarthrosis)) OR (Osteoarthroses)) OR (Arthritis, Degenerative)) OR (Arthritides, Degenerative)) OR (Degenerative Arthritides)) OR (Degenerative Arthritis)) OR (Arthrosis)) OR (Arthroses)) OR (Osteoarthrosis Deformans)) OR ("Osteoarthritis"[Mesh]))) AND (randomized controlled trial[Publication Type] OR randomized[Title/Abstract] OR placebo[Title/Abstract]).

We also manually checked the bibliographies of the identified articles, including relevant reviews and meta-analyses, to identify additional eligible studies. Furthermore, we searched three clinical trial registries (ClinicalTrials.gov, Controlled-trials.com, and Umin.ac.jp/ctr/index. The htm), as we allowed the inclusion of unpublished clinical studies.

Selection criteria

We included studies in this systematic review and meta-analysis based on the following criteria: (1) patients: patients diagnosed with KOA based on the criteria described by the American College of Rheumatology; (2) intervention: treatment with anti-IL-1 therapeutics; (3) comparison: treatment with placebo, saline, or no treatment; (4) outcomes: at least 1 of the following outcomes: the Western Ontario and McMaster Universities Osteoarthritis Index (WOMAC) total score, WOMAC subscores (pain, function, and stiffness), the visual analogue scale (VAS) score for pain, the pain and function subitem scores of the Knee Injury and Osteoarthritis Outcome Score (KOOS), and adverse events (defined as local and systemic reactions such as pain, stiffness, swelling, dizziness, headache, nausea, or infection); and (5) studies: RCTs. The following studies will be excluded: (1) other documents included due to expansion of search scope, such as retrospective research, review, or meta-analysis; (2) non-knee joint; (3) failed to obtain outcome indicators; (4) small sample size: less than 5 participants in intervention arms; and (5) non-RCT.

Selection of studies

EndNote (Version 20; Clarivate Analytics) was used to manage the selection of studies, including duplicate removal. Two reviewers (R.L. and Q.Z.) independently carried out the initial search, removed duplicate records, screened the titles and abstracts for relevance, and classified each study as included, excluded. We resolved disagreements by consensus. If no agreement was met, a third review author (G.Q.) acted as arbiter.

Data extraction

Data were extracted by 2 reviewers (R.L. and Q.Z.), input into a standardized electronic form, and checked by a third reviewer (G.Q.). Disagreements were resolved through discussion before the analyses were performed. The following data were extracted: first author, year of publication, country, company, number of participants, age, sex, body mass index (BMI), severity of OA, intervention, method of administration, and outcome data. Predefined primary outcomes were WOMAC pain and function scores, the VAS score for pain, the pain and function subitem scores of the KOOS, any AE, serious AEs (SAEs), and discontinuations due to AEs. An AE that was life-threatening, disabling, led to hospitalization or death, or led to a birth defect or congenital anomaly was classified as a SAE. It was classified as discontinuation due to AEs when patient dropped out of the trial or patient was withdrawn from the trial at the judgement of the investigator due to any AE. When the same patients were reported in several publications, we retained only the latest study to avoid the duplication of information. Because of the different follow-up times of these identified studies, we pooled and calculated data from around a similar time frame. Since the shortest follow-up among these identified studies is 3 months, data from follow-up in the second or third month were merged.

Risk of bias assessment

Two reviewers (R.L. and Q.Z.) used the Cochrane Risk of Bias tool to assess the risk of bias in the RCTs. Each study was reviewed and scored as having a high, low, or unclear risk of bias according to the following domains: random sequence generation, allocation concealment, blinding of participants and personnel, blinding of outcome assessment, incomplete outcome data, selective reporting, and other bias. Discrepancies between the reviewers were resolved by discussion until consensus was achieved.

Data analysis and statistical methods

We analysed the results of the studies using RevMan 5.4 (Cochrane Collaboration, Oxford, UK). Results of dichotomous data were presented as risk ratios (RR) with the corresponding 95% confidence intervals (95% CI). An RR greater than 1.0 indicated a beneficial effect of anti-IL-1 therapeutics. Results of continuous data were presented as mean differences (MD) between the intervention and comparator groups with the corresponding 95% CIs. Since pain and function were measured by different scales, we calculated

Yu *et al. Journal of Orthopaedic Surgery and Research* (2023) 18:100

standardized mean differences (SMD) with the corresponding 95% CIs instead. For the calculation of SMD, we divided the MD by the standard deviation, resulting in a unit-less measure of treatment effect. SMDs less than zero indicated a beneficial effect of the anti-interleukin-1 therapeutics. As described by Cohen, an SMD of 0.2 indicates a small beneficial effect, 0.5 a medium effect, and 0.8 a large effect in favour of anti-interleukin-1 therapeutics [50]. Statistical heterogeneity was assessed using a standard chi-square test and was considered significant at $p < 0.05$. Pooled data were analysed using a random effects model because we assumed that there is heterogeneity caused by factors other than chance. The overall effect size is shown in forest plots. We stratified the analyses according to the mechanism of action to understand the effects of different anti-IL-1 therapeutics on pain and function and the AEs associated with treatment.

Results

Literature search

Figure 1 shows the process of the study selection and inclusion. A total of 728 potential studies were identified with the initial search strategy. A total of 10 studies were obtained after the manual reference review, and one unpublished study was retrieved from ClinicalTrials.gov. After the examination of the titles and abstracts, 15 eligible studies were assessed for potential inclusion. After reviewing the full texts, 12 RCTs were included in the meta-analysis [51–62].

Study characteristics

The detailed information of the included studies and the baseline characteristics of the included patients are presented in Tables 1 and 2, respectively. The anti-IL-1 therapeutics evaluated in the literature could be divided into the following three categories based on their mechanism

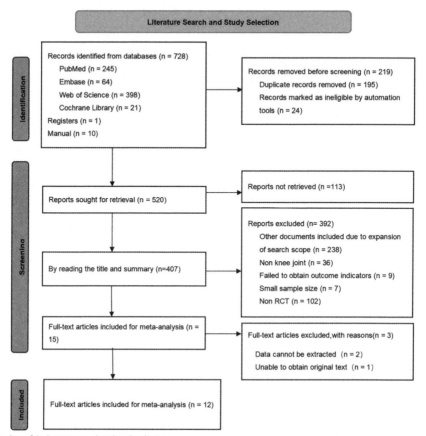

Fig. 1 Flow chart of the literature search and study selection

Yu *et al. Journal of Orthopaedic Surgery and Research*　　(2023) 18:100

Table 1 Detailed information of the included studies

Study and year	Type	Country	Company	Medicine	Intervention	Follow-up, weeks	Group	Subgroup§	Outcomes‡
Fleischmann 2019 [51]	RCT	USA	AbbVie Inc	ABT981(IL-1 antibody)	SC, once every 2 weeks, lasting for 50 weeks	52	25 mg 100 mg 200 mg	Subgroup 1 Subgroup 2 Subgroup 3	①②⑥
Cohen 2011 [52]	RCT	USA	Amgen Inc	AMG 108 (IL-1 Ras)	SC, once every 4 weeks, lasting for 12 weeks IV, once every 4 weeks, lasting for 12 weeks SC, once every 4 weeks, lasting for 12 weeks	12	75 mg 300 mg 100 mg 300 mg 300 mg	Subgroup 1 Subgroup 2 Subgroup 3 Subgroup 4 Subgroup5	⑥
Baltzer 2009 [53]	Multicentre enter RCT	Germany	NA	Orthokine† (IL-1 Ras)	IA, twice a week, lasting for 3 weeks	26	NA	Subgroup 1	①②⑤⑥
Yang 2008 [54]	RCT	Netherlands	NA	Orthokine† (IL-1 Ras)	IA on days 0, 3, 7, 10, 14 and 21	48	NA	Subgroup 1	③④⑤
Wang 2017 [55]	RCT	USA	AbbVie Inc	ABT-981 (IL-1 antibody)	SC, once every 1 week, lasting for 8 weeks SC, once every 4 weeks, lasting for 12 weeks	16.7 18.1	0.3 mg/kg 1 mg/kg 3 mg/kg 3 mg/kg	Subgroup 1 Subgroup 2 Subgroup 3 Subgroup 4	⑥
Chevalier 2009 [56]	Multicentre enter RCT	France	Amgen Inc	Anakinra (IL-1 Ras)	Single IA	12	50 mg 150 mg	Subgroup 1 Subgroup 2	⑤⑥
Kosloski 2016 [57]	RCT	USA	AbbVie Inc	ABT-981(IL-1 antibody)	SC, once every 2 weeks, lasting for 8 weeks SC, once every 4 weeks, lasting for 12 weeks	18	0.3 mg/kg 1 mg/kg 3 mg/kg 3 mg/kg	Subgroup 1 Subgroup 2 Subgroup 3 Subgroup 4	⑥
NCT01160822 2012[58]	RCT	USA	Novartis Inc	Canaki-numab (IL-1 antibody)	Single IA Single IA of canaki-numab + oral placebo twice a day (control group: placebo + placebo), lasting for 12 weeks	18	150 mg 300 mg 600 mg 600 mg Canaki-numab + placebo	Subgroup 1 Subgroup 2 Subgroup 3 Subgroup 4	⑥
Brahmachari 2009 [59]	RCT	India	NA	Diacerein(IL-1 inhibitor)	Oral, once a day for the first 10 days, 50 mg after meals, lasting for 8 weeks	12	NA	Subgroup 1	②⑤⑥
Pelletier 2000 [60]	Multicentre enter RCT	France	Les Laboratoires Negma	Diacerein(IL-1 inhibitor)	Oral twice a day for 16 weeks	12	50 mg 100 mg 150 mg	Subgroup 1 Subgroup 2 Subgroup 3	①②⑤⑥
Pham 2004 [61]	Multicentre enter RCT	France	NA	Diacerein(IL-1 inhibitor)	Oral twice a day for 12 weeks	48	NA	Subgroup 1	⑤⑥

Yu *et al. Journal of Orthopaedic Surgery and Research*   (2023) 18:100

Table 1 (continued)

Study and year	Type	Country	Company	Medicine	Intervention	Follow-up, weeks	Group	Subgroup§	Outcomes‡
Pavelka 2007 [62]	Multicentre enter RCT	Czech	TRB Chemedica and Glynn Brothers Chemicals	Diacerein(IL-1 inhibitor)	Oral twice a day for 12 weeks	24	NA	Subgroup 1	②⑥

* *RCT* randomized controlled trial; *SC* subcutaneous injection; *IV* intravenous injection; *IA* intra-articular injection; *WOMAC* Western Ontario and McMaster Universities Osteoarthritis Index; *KOOS* Knee Injury and Osteoarthritis Outcome Score; *VAS* visual analogue scale; and *NA* not available Universities Osteoarthritis Index

† Orthokine: Orthokine is the trade name of autologous-conditioned serum (ACS)

‡ Data extraction results of outcomes: ① WOMAC pain score; ② WOMAC function score; ③ KOOS pain score; ④ KOOS function score; ⑤ VAS score; and ⑥ adverse events

§ Due to the limited number of studies, we named and grouped the research projects in different ways according to the original research

Baseline characteristics of studies included in the meta-analysis

of action. Placebo was used as control groups in all 12 studies, but only three of them clearly informed that physiological saline was used as placebo [53, 54, 61], and others had not explained what was used as placebo. The sample size of the studies ranged from 36 to 480, for a total of 2192 knees, including 1361 knees in the anti-IL-1 therapeutics group and 831 knees in the placebo group.

Risk of bias

The results of the risk of bias assessment are summarized in Fig. 2. Among the 12 studies, 7 studies were judged to have a high risk of bias [55, 57–62], and 5 were found to have a moderate risk of bias [51–54, 56]. An adequate randomized sequence was generated in 9 studies [53–57, 59–62], appropriate allocation concealment was reported in 4 studies [54, 56, 58, 59], the blinding of participants was clear in 7 studies [54–56, 58, 59, 61, 62], the blinding of outcome assessors was reported in 6 studies [53–56, 58, 62], outcome data were complete in 9 studies [51–53, 55, 56, 59–62], 6 studies had no selective reporting [51–54, 56, 58], and 5 studies had no other bias [53, 59–62].

Knee pain scores

Following anti-IL-1 or control treatment, four studies [51, 53, 60, 62] assessed pain scores with the WOMAC, and four studies [54, 56, 59, 61] assessed pain scores with the VAS. We found a statistically significant pain decrease in the anti-IL-1 therapeutic group compared with the control group (SMD $= -0.38$, 95% CI: -0.62 to -0.14; $p < 0.001$; $I^2 = 77\%$, Fig. 3). The details of the subgroup analyses are presented in Fig. 4.

Knee function scores

Following anti-IL-1 or control treatment, five studies [51, 53, 54, 59, 60, 62] assessed function scores with the WOMAC, and one study [54] assessed function scores with the KOOS. Significant improvement in knee function was found in the anti-IL-1 therapeutic group compared with the control group (SMD $= -1.11$, 95% CI: -1.82 to -0.40; $p = 0.002$; $I^2 = 96\%$, Fig. 5). Details of the subgroup analyses are presented in Fig. 6.

Safety of biological agents in the treatment of OA
Any AE

A total of 11 studies provided data on the incidence of any AE. Among all AEs, infections, injection site reactions and neutropenia were commonly observed in patients treated with IL-1 antibodies. Headache and upper respiratory tract infections were more frequent in OA patients treated with IL-1 Ras. More patients treated with the IL-1 inhibitor had knee pain, respiratory system disorders, diarrhoea, skin disorders, and gastrointestinal disorders. Overall, the incidence of any AE was significantly different between the anti-IL-1 therapeutic group and the placebo group (RR $= 1.02$, 95% CI $= 0.88$–1.18, $p < 0.001$, $I2 = 76\%$) (Fig. 7). Details of the subgroup analyses are presented in Fig. 8.

Serious AEs

The SAEs in patients treated with IL-1 Ras included haemorrhagic diarrhoea, pneumonia, pancreatitis, and Staphylococcus infection. Serious infection, malignancy, fracture, and injury were observed in RCTs of IL-1 antibodies, but no serious complications were reported with IL-1 inhibitor therapy. Notably, no significant difference was found between the anti-IL-1 therapeutic and placebo groups in terms of the incidence of SAEs (RR $= 0.43$, 95% CI $= 0.20$–0.92, $p = 0.90$, $I^2 = 0\%$) (Fig. 9). Compared with placebo, neither IL-1 Ras nor IL-1 antibodies were associated with any significantly increased incidence of SAEs (Fig. 10).

附录 2　论文范例

Yu *et al. Journal of Orthopaedic Surgery and Research*　　　(2023) 18:100　　　　　　　　　　　　　　　　　　　　　Page 7 of 16

Table 2 Baseline characteristics of the included patients*

Study and year	Subgroup	Sample size, n		Female, n (%)		Age, y (M±SD)		BMI, kg/m² (M±SD)		Kellgren and Lawrence grading scale, n (%)				Course of OA, y (M±SD)	
		Treat	Control	Treat	Control	Treat	Control	Treat	Control	Treat Grade II	Treat Grade III	Control Grade II	Control Grade III	Treat	Control
Fleischmann 2019 [51]	Subgroup 1	89	85	63 (70.8)	52 (61.2)	61.6±7.5	59.5±8.9	28.7±3.8	28.6±3.6	57 (64.0)	32 (36.0)	53 (62.4)	32 (37.6)	7.6±9.0	7.9±8.0
	Subgroup 2	85		53 (62.4)		60.2±8.2		29.0±3.5		52 (61.2)	33 (38.8)			7.9±8.7	
	Subgroup 3	88		57 (64.8)		59.1±10.3		28.7±3.5		56 (63.6)	32 (36.4)			8.7±8.6	
Cohen 2011 [52]	Subgroup 1	12	16	9 (75)	10 (63)	62.3	60.8	30.9	30.4	4 (33)	5 (42)	4 (25)	10 (63)	10	9.6
	Subgroup 2	12		5 (42)		59.6		29.8		5 (42)	7 (58)			6.6	
	Subgroup 3	12		11 (92)		61.1		30.8		3 (25)	6 (50)			6.9	
	Subgroup 4	12		7 (58)		62.8		31.9		7 (58)	4 (33)			10.2	
	Subgroup5	80	80	54 (68)	54 (68)	61.3	60.1	32	31.9	40 (50)	39 (49)	30 (38)	46 (58)	6.1	6.1
Baltzer 2009 [53]	Subgroup 1	134	107	65 (48.5)	68 (63.6)	53.8±12.2	60.3±10.7	NA	NA	NA	NA	NA	NA	NA	NA
Yang 2008 [54]	Subgroup 1	73	67	49 (61)	43 (59)	54±11	53±11	27±5	28±14	NA	NA	NA	NA	NA	NA
Wang 2017 [55]	Subgroup 1	7	6	5 (71.4)	5 (83.3)	61.3±5.1	60.0±5.9	27.6±4.4	28.4±2.3	NA	NA	NA	NA	NA	NA
	Subgroup 2	7		5 (71.4)		62.6±3.6		26.4±1.1		NA	NA			NA	
	Subgroup 3	7		5 (71.4)		61.4±5.0		27.3±2.9		NA	NA			NA	
	Subgroup 4	7		7 (100)		60.0±6.1		29.3±3.0		NA	NA			NA	
Chevalier 2009 [56]	Subgroup 1	34	2	17 (50)	2 (100)	63.3±9.8	55.0±1.4	NA	8.7±0.5	3 (4)	18 (53)	27 (39)	42 (61)	8.1±9.8	6.0±6.2
	Subgroup 2	67	69	46 (69)	44 (64)	62.6±9.4	62.2±10.0	NA	NA	24 (37)	39 (58)	NA	NA	5.2±5.7	
Kosloski 2016 [57]	Subgroup 1	7	8	24 (86)	7 (88)	61.3±11.85	58.8±9.63	NA	NA	NA	NA	NA	NA	NA	NA
	Subgroup 2	7		NA		NA		NA		NA	NA			NA	
	Subgroup 3	7		NA		NA		NA		NA	NA			NA	
	Subgroup 4	7		NA		NA		NA		NA	NA			NA	
NCT01160822 2012	Subgroup 1	6	5	7 (88)	2 (40)	58.3±12.79	57.8±7.76	NA	NA	NA	NA	NA	NA	NA	NA
	Subgroup 2	7		4 (57.1)		61.0±9.63		NA		NA	NA			NA	
	Subgroup 3	6		2 (33.3)		64.2±10.68		NA		NA	NA			NA	
	Subgroup 4	45	47	31 (68.9)	31 (66)	61.4±8.96	60.3±9.71	NA	NA	NA	NA	NA	NA	NA	NA
Brahmachari 2009 [59]	Subgroup 1	28	27	26 (92.8)	20 (74)	45.5±10.52	53±11.85	25.3±3.63	20±3.70	10	18	12	15	3.5±6.0	2.0±3.3
Pelletier 2000 [60]	Subgroup 1	126	124	105 (83.3)	98 (79)	62.95±8.41	64.5±8.65	31.63±5.50	31.05±5.35	NA	NA	NA	NA	7.8±7.18	8.0±7.41
	Subgroup 2	110		83 (75.5)		64.22±8.02		31.73±6.21		NA	NA			8.1±6.42	
	Subgroup 3	120		96 (80)		62.27±10.18		30.99±5.88		NA	NA			7.8±6.99	
Pham 2004 [61]	Subgroup 1	85	85	59 (69.4)	52 (61.2)	64.5±7.8	64.9±7.7	NA	NA	12 (14)	66 (79)	19 (23)	60 (72)	NA	NA
Pavelka 2007 [62]	Subgroup 1	82	83	67 (81.7)	64 (77.1)	63.5±8.39	63.8±8.09	28.7±4.1	29.1±3.9	54 (65.9)	27 (32.9)	48 (57.8)	35 (42.2)	6.87±6.16	6.13±5.61

* *BMI* body mass index; *M* mean; *NA* not available; *SD* standard deviation; and continuous data are depicted in M when SD is not available

Yu et al. Journal of Orthopaedic Surgery and Research   (2023) 18:100

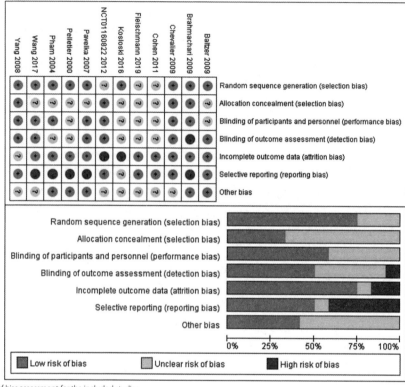

Fig. 2 Risk of bias assessment for the included studies

Discontinuation due to AEs

The number of patients discontinued due to AEs was extracted from 9 studies with the data available. No significant difference was found in the incidence of discontinuations due to AEs between the experimental groups and the control group (RR = 0.94, 95% CI = 0.60–1.47, $p = 1.00$, $I^2 = 0\%$) (Fig. 11). Compared with placebo, none of the three types of anti-IL-1 therapeutics were associated with any significantly increased incidence of discontinuations due to AEs (Fig. 12).

Discussion

This meta-analysis comprehensively investigated the efficacy and safety of anti-IL-1 therapeutics, including IL-1 antibodies, an IL-1 inhibitor, and IL-1 Ras, in patients with KOA. The pooled results indicated that anti-IL-1 therapeutics were significantly superior to placebo in terms of pain relief and functional improvement. The incidence of any AE was higher following treatment with anti-IL-1 therapeutics; however, no significant difference in SAEs or discontinuations due to AEs was found

compared with placebo. Subgroup analyses showed that IL-1 antibodies and the IL-1 inhibitor provided superior pain relief and functional improvement, whereas IL-1 Ras did not. However, the IL-1 inhibitor increased the incidence of any AE but not of SAEs or discontinuations due to AEs. IL-1 antibodies and IL-1 Ras showed no difference in safety compared with placebo.

To update the anti-IL-1 therapeutic evidence in the treatment of KOA, we included 12 RCTs covering three anti-IL-1 therapeutic categories based on the mechanism of action: ABT981, AMH108, and canakinumab were reported in four studies as IL-1 antibodies [51, 55, 57, 58]; Orthokine and Anakinra were reported in four studies as IL-1 Ras [52–54, 56]; and diacerein was reported in four studies as an IL-1 inhibitor [59–62]. Compared with previous studies that were either narrative reviews or meta-analyses involving only some anti-IL-1 therapeutics [46–48], the present work comprehensively evaluated the efficacy and safety of the three main anti-IL-1 therapeutics, including IL-1 antibodies, IL-1 Ras, and an IL-1 inhibitor. Considering

附录 2　论文范例

Yu *et al. Journal of Orthopaedic Surgery and Research*　　(2023) 18:100

Page 9 of 16

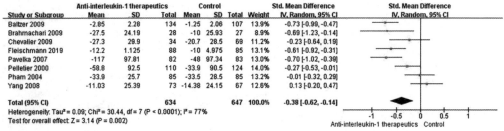

Fig. 3 Knee pain score results

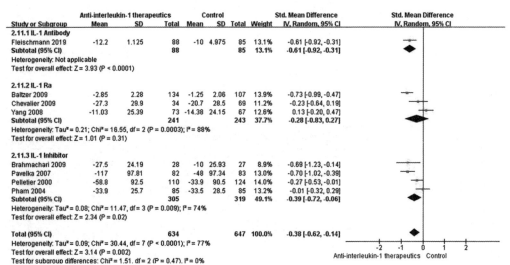

Fig. 4 Knee pain score results by subgroup

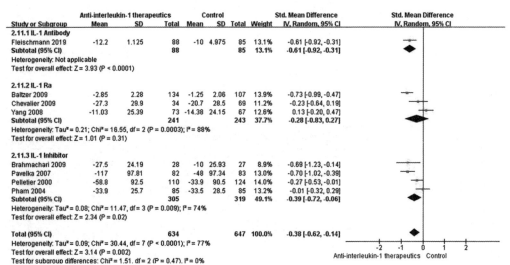

Fig. 5 Knee function score results

that all of the included trials were double-blinded randomized placebo-controlled trials, our subgroup analyses according to the mechanism of action enabled indirect comparisons for these three main anti-IL-1 therapeutic categories.

The antagonism of IL-1 in the treatment of OA as well as the potential pathways has been continuously discovered [63–65]. The study conducted by Chevalier [66] indicated that IL-1 can increase the production of matrix metalloproteinase (MMP) and inhibit the synthesis of

Yu *et al. Journal of Orthopaedic Surgery and Research*   (2023) 18:100

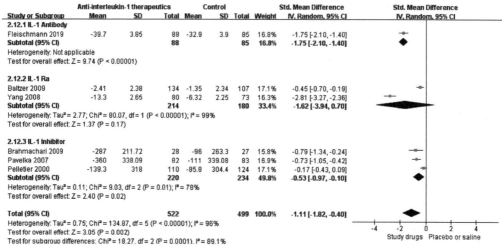

Fig. 6 Knee function score results by subgroup

Fig. 7 Results for any AE

type II collagen and proteoglycans. MMP is one of the major enzymes in the degradation of cartilage extracellular matrix components, and type II collagen and proteoglycans are important intermediate substances that can promote chondrocyte differentiation. Honourati et al. reported that IL1-β can enhance vascular endothelial growth factor (VEGF) secretion to varying degrees through dedifferentiated OA chondrocytes. Several studies have shown that reducing IL-1 by different means can inhibit the inflammatory response caused by IL-1 in human OA chondrocytes [67–70]. Therefore, the IL-1 pathway is a promising target for the treatment of patients with OA. The three types of anti-interleukin-1 therapeutics, including IL-1 antibodies, IL-1 Ras, and IL-1 inhibitors, are all therapeutic agents that interfere

with the IL-1 pathway. IL-1 antibodies are a kind of therapeutic human dual variable domain immunoglobulins capable of potently neutralizing human IL-1α and/ or IL-1β [71]. The interleukin-1 receptor antagonist (IL-1Ra) is a member of the IL-1 family that binds to IL-1 receptors, which is an important anti-inflammatory protein in arthritis [72]. IL-1 inhibitor is defined as a kind of purified compound which can inhibit the production and activity of interleukin 1 [61].

Since different scales (the WOMAC and VAS for pain evaluation, the WOMAC and KOOS scales for function evaluation) were used in the studies included, we calculated the SMD for each study using Cohen's d method. According to our results, anti-IL-1 therapeutics provided statistically significant effects on pain relief and

Yu *et al. Journal of Orthopaedic Surgery and Research*　(2023) 18:100

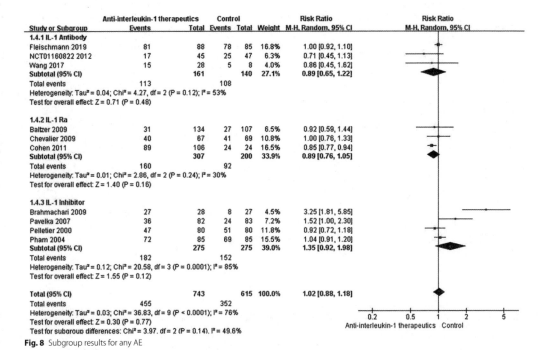

Fig. 8 Subgroup results for any AE

Fig. 9 Results for SAEs

functional improvement. The results of subgroup analyses according to the mechanism of action showed that IL-1 antibodies and the IL-1 inhibitor were both associated with significantly higher pain relief and functional improvement than placebo, but IL-1 Ras were not. Several studies have been reported to evaluate the efficacy of anti-IL-1 therapeutics in KOA. A systematic review indicated that IL-1 Ra may be an effective adjunct for those unresponsive to traditional intra-articular therapies [46], which is consistent with our results. However, another meta-analysis indicated that IL-1 antibodies led to no

improvement in pain or function compared to placebo [48]. The number of research articles on anti-IL-1 therapeutics in KOA is not enough to reach a consensus on the efficacy of IL for KOA, and more randomized controlled trials and meta-analysis are necessary to update the anti-IL-1 therapeutic evidence in the treatment of KOA.

With respect to the safety of anti-IL-1 therapeutics, the results of further subgroup analyses showed that the IL-1 inhibitor was associated with a higher incidence of any AE, whereas IL-1 antibodies and IL-1 Ras were not. The common AEs in the treatment of IL-1

Yu et al. Journal of Orthopaedic Surgery and Research   (2023) 18:100

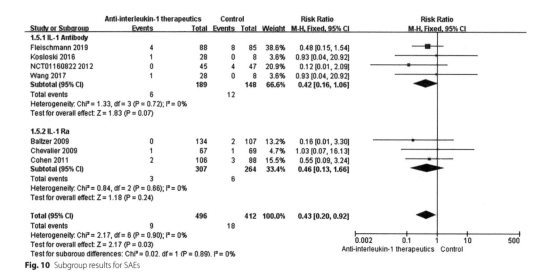

Fig. 10 Subgroup results for SAEs

Fig. 11 Results for discontinuations due to AEs

inhibitors were pain, respiratory system disorders, diarrhoea, skin disorders, and gastrointestinal disorders. These adverse events are self-limited and can resolve following adequate rest. According to the results of the subgroup analyses, IL-1 antibodies, IL-1 Ras, and the IL-1 inhibitor were not associated with a significant difference in SAEs or discontinuations due to AEs compared with placebo. Because of the small number of studies included, we did not perform a further analysis on the effect of different interventions on any AE, SAEs, or discontinuations due to AEs. Therefore, the safety of the IL-1 inhibitor reveals the need for further investigations and great caution in upcoming trials. Contrary to the IL-1 inhibitor, IL-1 antibodies and IL-1 Ras showed favourable tolerability in the treatment of

KOA, but attention should still be given to the risk of infection, even if there are no safety concerns.

There is substantial heterogeneity surrounding the treatment effects reported, even after splitting the analyses in subgroups. We consider several reasons to explain this phenomenon. First, different medicines were used in different studies even in the same subgroup (Table.1). IL-1 antibodies included two medicines: ABT981, AMH108, and canakinumab. IL-1 Ras included three medicines: AMG 108, Orthokine, and Anakinra. Second, dosing, method, and/or frequency of administration were inconsistent (Table 1). Dosing varied from 25 to 600 mg. Subcutaneous injection, intravenous injection, and oral were applied in different studies. Frequency varied from twice a day to once every 4 weeks. Third, the pain and

Yu et al. Journal of Orthopaedic Surgery and Research   (2023) 18:100

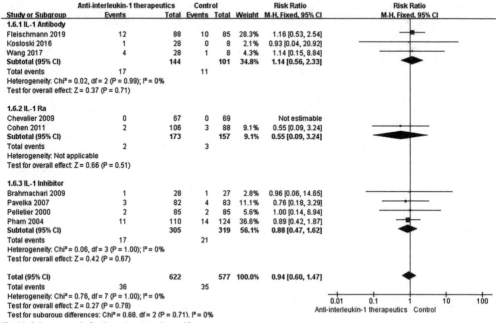

Fig. 12 Subgroup results for discontinuations due to AEs

function outcome were assessed by different scales: the WOMAC and VAS for pain evaluation, the WOMAC and KOOS scales for function evaluation. Besides, baseline characteristics of the included patients in the same subgroups were also inconsistent. All of above reasons may contribute to substantial heterogeneity after splitting the analyses in subgroups. But limited by the small number of studies included, we could not perform a further subgroups analysis for above factors.

This study has several strengths. Our extensive literature search makes it seems unlikely to miss the clinical RCT associated with this study and the latest RCT for inclusion in the field to date. Trial selection and data extraction, including quality assessment, were performed independently by 2 authors and were discussed with a third senior orthopaedic specialist, thus minimizing bias and the occurrence of transcriptional errors. The highlight is that, unlike other meta-analyses that included studies about only one of the mechanism of anti-IL-1 therapeutics, our study included the latest RCTs about three mechanisms of anti-IL-1 therapeutics, thus providing the most comprehensive update on the effectiveness and safety of anti-IL-1 therapeutics for the treatment of KOA. Only RCTs were included; therefore, by excluding observational studies, we removed the inherent selection

bias associated with that study design. A detailed assessment of the methodological quality of the included studies was performed. In addition, we performed subgroup analyses according to the different mechanisms of action of anti-IL-1 therapeutics, thus observing the effect of the IL-1 inhibitor, IL-1 antibodies, and IL-1 Ras on the target outcome separately and overcoming the limitations of the previous systematic evaluation.

Limitations

This study has several limitations. First, similar to most systematic evaluations, our study was limited by the quality of the included RCTs. Most trials were of poor methodological quality or showed selective reporting. Only four trials [54, 56, 58, 59] described the method of allocation concealment. The potential risk of bias weakened our ability to draw conclusions regarding the treatment effects. Second, none of the included studies reported on knee survivorship, that is, the number of patients for whom anti-IL-1 therapeutics ultimately failed and thus went on to undergo total knee arthroplasty. Third, the studies included were heterogeneous in terms of dosage and intervention, which are factors that may lead to differing biological activity of anti-IL-1 therapeutics and thus different physiological responses in patients.

Yu et al. Journal of Orthopaedic Surgery and Research   (2023) 18:100

Additionally, the follow-up time among the included studies also varied, ranging from 12 to 52 weeks. Furthermore, there was no publication bias in this study. The authors had considered assessing publication bias by funnel plot once but we had not done it finally. As Sterne JAC, Sutton A J et al. thought, tests for funnel plot asymmetry should not be used when there are fewer than 10 studies in the meta-analysis because test power is usually too low to distinguish chance from real asymmetry [73]. There are only eight studies with knee pain outcome and only five studies with knee function score in our meta-analysis. These factors weakened our ability to draw conclusions on the effect of anti-IL-1 therapeutics compared with control treatment for KOA.

Conclusions

Our study updates the anti-IL-1 therapeutic evidence in the treatment of KOA. Anti-interleukin-1 therapeutics could relieve OA-related pain and improve function, but is probably associated with an increased risk of adverse events. Specially, the efficacy and safety of anti-IL-1 therapeutics varied according to the mechanism of action. IL-1 antibodies and an IL-1 inhibitor could relieve OA-related pain and improve function, whereas IL-1 Ras could not. IL-1 antibodies and IL-1 Ras were relatively safe options, but IL-1 inhibitors were associated with safety concerns. Due to the low quality of the studies and the limited data currently available, more high-quality RCTs are needed.

Abbreviations

IL-1 Ra	Interleukin-1 receptor antagonists
KOA	Knee osteoarthritis
RCT	Randomized controlled trial
AE	Adverse effect
SMD	Standardized mean difference
RR	Risk ratio
SAE	Serious adverse effect
CI	Confidence interval
OA	Osteoarthritis
NSAIDs	Nonsteroidal anti-inflammatory drugs
HA	Hyaluronic acid
IL	Interleukin
TNF	Tumour necrosis factor
NGF	Nerve growth factor
PRISMA	Preferred Reporting Items for Systematic Reviews and Meta-Analyses
MeSH	Medical Subject Headings
WOMAC	Western Ontario and McMaster Universities Osteoarthritis Index
VAS	Visual analogue scale
KOOS	Knee Injury and Osteoarthritis Outcome Score
BMI	Body mass index
I-V	Inverse-variance

Acknowledgements
Everyone who contributed significantly to this study has been listed.

Author contributions
R.L. and Q.Z. conducted a systematic literature search and extracted data from the included studies and assessed the risk of bias. G.Q. acted as arbiter when there were discrepancies. L.Y. analysed study data and was a major contributor in writing the manuscript. W.L. is responsible for ensuring that the descriptions are accurate and agreed by all authors. All authors read and approved the final manuscript.

Funding
The authors disclose the receipt of the following financial support for the research, authorship, and/or publication of this article: This work was supported by the Guangxi Natural Science Foundation (AD19245017), the Scientific Research Foundation of Guangxi University of Science and Technology(20Z13), the Scientific Research Foundation of Guangxi Health Commission (Z20211376), and the Scientific Research Foundation of Guangxi Health Commission (Z20190410).

Availability of data and materials
The data that support the findings of this study are available from the corresponding author upon reasonable request.

Declarations

Ethics approval and consent to participate
Not applicable.

Consent for publication
Not applicable.

Competing interests
The authors declare that they have no competing interests.

Author details
[1]The First Affiliated Hospital of Guangxi University of Science and Technology, Guangxi University of Science and Technology, 124 Yuejin Road, Liuzhou 545001, Guangxi Province, China.

Received: 22 October 2022   Accepted: 7 February 2023
Published online: 13 February 2023

References
1. Goldring SR, Goldring MB. Changes in the osteochondral unit during osteoarthritis: structure, function and cartilage-bone crosstalk. Nat Rev Rheumatol. 2016;12:632–44.
2. Felson DT, Zhang Y. An update on the epidemiology of knee and hip osteoarthritis with a view to prevention. Arthritis Rheum. 1998;41:1343–55.
3. Atabatie Fard MM, Malakimoghadmh Jafarzadeh, Fard MM. Comparison of the effect of avocado/soybean extract and crocin on pain intensity and radiographic changes in patients with knee osteoarthritis. J Complement Med Res. 2021;12(1):127–132.
4. Oliveira AMID, Peccin MS, Silva KNGd, Teixeira LEPDP, Trevisani VFM. Impacto dos exercícios na capacidade funcional e dor em pacientes com osteoartrite de joelhos: ensaio clínico randomizado. Rev Bras Reumatol. 2012;52:876–82.
5. Sayre EC, Li LC, Kopec JA, Esdaile JM, Bar S, Cibere J. The effect of disease site (knee, hip, hand, foot, lower back or neck) on employment reduction due to osteoarthritis. PLoS ONE. 2010;5: e10470.
6. Hutton I, Gamble G, McLean G, Butcher H, Gow P, Dalbeth N. Obstacles to action in arthritis: a community case-control study. Int J Rheum Dis. 2009;12:107–17.
7. Carr AJ, Robertsson O, Graves S, Price AJ, Arden NK, Judge A, et al. Knee replacement. Lancet. 2012;379:1331–40.
8. Richmond J, Hunter D, Irrgang J, Jones MH, Snyder-Mackler L, Van Durme D, et al. American academy of orthopaedic surgeons clinical practice guideline on the treatment of osteoarthritis (OA) of the knee. J Bone Jt Surg Am. 2010;92:990–3.
9. Katz JN, Arant KR, Loeser RF. Diagnosis and treatment of hip and knee osteoarthritis: a review. JAMA. 2021;325:568–78.
10. Bijlsma JWJ, Berenbaum F, Lafeber FPJG. Osteoarthritis: an update with relevance for clinical practice. Lancet. 2011;377:2115–26.

Yu *et al. Journal of Orthopaedic Surgery and Research*　　(2023) 18:100

11. Wang SY, Olson-Kellogg B, Shamliyan TA, Choi JY, Ramakrishnan R, Kane RL. Physical therapeutic interventions for knee pain secondary to osteoarthritis: a systematic review. Ann Intern Med. 2012;157:632–44.

12. McAlindon TE, Bannuru RR, Sullivan MC, Arden NK, Berenbaum F, Bierma-Zeinstra SM, et al. OARSI guidelines for the non-surgical management of knee osteoarthritis. Osteoarthr Cartil. 2014;22:363–88.

13. Jevsevar DS. Treatment of osteoarthritis of the knee: evidence-based guideline, 2nd edition. J Am Acad Orthop Surg. 2013;21:571–6.

14. Sheean AJ, Anz AW, Bradley JP. Platelet-rich plasma: fundamentals and clinical applications. Arthroscopy. 2021;37:2732–4.

15. de Andrade MAP, Campos TVDO, Abreu-e-Silva GMD. Supplementary methods in the nonsurgical treatment of osteoarthritis. Arthroscopy. 2015;31:785–92.

16. Jüni P, Nartey L, Reichenbach S, Sterchi R, Dieppe PA, Egger M. Risk of cardiovascular events and rofecoxib: cumulative meta-analysis. Lancet. 2004;364:2021–9.

17. Machado GC, Maher CG, Ferreira PH, Pinheiro MB, Lin C-WC, Day RO, et al. Efficacy and safety of paracetamol for spinal pain and osteoarthritis: systematic review and meta-analysis of randomised placebo controlled trials. BMJ (Clinical researched). 2015;350:h1225.

18. Leopoldino AO, Machado GC, Ferreira PH, Pinheiro MB, Day R, McLachlan AJ, et al. Paracetamol versus placebo for knee and hip osteoarthritis. Cochrane Database Syst Rev. 2019;2:CD013273.

19. Zhang W, Moskowitz RW, Nuki G, Abramson S, Altman RD, Arden N, et al. OARSI recommendations for the management of hip and knee osteoarthritis, part I: critical appraisal of existing treatment guidelines and systematic review of current research evidence. Osteoarthritis Cartilage. 2007;15:981–1000.

20. Jordan KM, Arden NK, Doherty M, Bannwarth B, Bijlsma JWJ, Dieppe P, et al. EULAR recommendations 2003: an evidence based approach to the management of knee osteoarthritis: report of a task force of the standing committee for international clinical studies including therapeutic trials (ESCISIT). Ann Rheum Dis. 2003;62:1145–55.

21. Hernandez-Diaz S, Varas-Lorenzo C, Rodriguez LAG. Non-steroidal antiinflammatory drugs and the risk of acute myocardial infarction. Basic Clin Pharmacol Toxicol. 2006;98:266–74.

22. Porcheret M, Jordan K, Jinks C. Primary care treatment of knee pain a survey in older adults. Rheumatology. 2007;46:1694–700.

23. Dwyer T, Chahal J. Editorial commentary: injections for knee osteoarthritis: doc, you gotta help me! Arthroscopy. 2021;37:1288–9.

24. Kalso E, Aldington DJ, Moore RA. Drugs for neuropathic pain. BMJ. 2013;347: f7339.

25. Turk DC, Wilson HD, Cahana A. Treatment of chronic non-cancer pain. Lancet. 2011;377:2226–35.

26. Wassilew GI, Lehnigk U, Duda GN, Taylor WR, Matziolis G, Dynybil C. The expression of proinflammatory cytokines and matrix metalloproteinases in the synovial membranes of patients with osteoarthritis compared with traumatic knee disorders. Arthroscopy. 2010;26:1096–104.

27. Baliga VP, Jagiasi JD, Arun Kumar MS, Sankaralingam K, Veerappan V, Bolmall CS. 562 efficacy safety and tolerability of diacerein MR 100mg vs Diacerein 50mg in adult patients with osteoarthritis of the knee. Osteoarthr Cartil. 2010;18:S252.

28. Miller RE, Miller RJ, Malfait AM. Osteoarthritis joint pain: the cytokine connection. Cytokine. 2017;70:185–93.

29. Montagnoli C, Tiribuzi R, Crispoltoni L, Pistilli A, Stabile AM, Manfreda F, et al. β-NGF and β-NGF receptor upregulation in blood and synovial fluid in osteoarthritis. Biol Chem. 2017;398:1045–54.

30. Kapoor M, Martel-Pelletier J, Lajeunesse D, Pelletier JP, Fahmi H. Role of proinflammatory cytokines in the pathophysiology of osteoarthritis. Nat Rev Rheumatol. 2010;7:33–42.

31. Mantovani A, Dinarello CA, Molgora M, Garlanda C. Interleukin-1 and related cytokines in the regulation of inflammation and immunity. Immunity. 2019;50:778–95.

32. Boraschi D, Italiani P, Weil S, Martin MU. The family of the interleukin-1 receptors. Immunol Rev. 2017;281:197–232.

33. Jotanovic Z, Mihelic R, Sestan B, Dembic Z. Role of interleukin-1 inhibitors in osteoarthritis. Drugs Aging. 2012;29:343–58.

34. Theoleyre S, Wittrant Y, Tat SK, Fortun Y, Redini F, Heymann D. The molecular triad OPG/RANK/RANKL: involvement in the orchestration of pathophysiological bone remodeling. Cytokine Growth Factor Rev. 2004;15:457–75.

35. Liu XH, Kirschenbaum A, Yao S, Levine AC. The role of the interleukin-6/gp130 signaling pathway in bone metabolism. Vitam Horm. 2006;74:341–55.

36. Massicotte F, Lajeunesse D, Benderdour M, Pelletier JP, Hilal G, Duval N, et al. Can altered production of interleukin-1β, interleukin-6, transforming growth factor-β and prostaglandin E2 by isolated human subchondral osteoblasts identify two subgroups of osteoarthritic patients? Osteoarthr Cartil. 2002;10:491–500.

37. Paschos NK. Editorial commentary: Could biological treatments be the game-changing factor for osteoarthritis? Arthroscopy. 2019;35:2434–5.

38. Chahla J, Mandelbaum BR. Biological treatment for osteoarthritis of the knee: moving from bench to bedside—current practical concepts. Arthroscopy. 2018;34:1719–29.

39. Na HS, Park JS, Cho KH, Kwon JY, Choi JW, Jhun J, et al. Interleukin-1-interleukin-17 signaling axis induces cartilage destruction and promotes experimental osteoarthritis. Front Immunol. 2020;11:730.

40. Chien SY, Tsai CH, Liu SC, Huang CC, Lin TH, Yang YZ, et al. Noggin inhibits IL-1β and BMP-2 expression, and attenuates cartilage degeneration and subchondral bone destruction in experimental osteoarthritis. Cells. 2020;9:927.

41. Guan YJ, Li J, Yang X, Du S, Ding J, Gao Y, et al. Evidence that miR-146a attenuates aging- and trauma-induced osteoarthritis by inhibiting Notch 1, IL-6, and IL-1 mediated catabolism. Aging Cell. 2018;17:e12752.

42. Zhang X, Mao Z, Yu C. Suppression of early experimental osteoarthritis by gene transfer of interleukin-1 receptor antagonist and interleukin-10. J Orthop Res. 2004;22:742–50.

43. Pelletier JP, Caron JP, Evans C, Robbins PD, Georgescu HI, Jovanovic D, et al. In vivo suppression of early experimental osteoarthritis by interleukin-1 receptor antagonist using gene therapy. Arthritis Rheum. 1997;40:1012–9.

44. Caron JP, Fernandes JC, Martel-Pelletier J, Tardif G, Mineau F, Geng C, et al. Chondroprotective effect of intraarticular injections of interleukin-1 receptor antagonist in experimental osteoarthritis. Suppression of collagenase-1 expression. Arthritis Rheum. 1996;39:1535–44.

45. Wang BW, Jiang Y, Yao ZL, Chen PS, Yu B, Wang SN. Aucubin protects chondrocytes against IL-1β-induced apoptosis in vitro and inhibits osteoarthritis in mice model. Drug Des Dev Ther. 2019;13:3529–38.

46. Ajrawat P, Dwyer T, Chahal J. Autologous interleukin 1 receptor antagonist blood-derived products for knee osteoarthritis: a systematic review. Arthroscopy. 2019;35:2211–21.

47. Meng F, Li H, Feng H, Long H, Yang Z, Li J, et al. Efficacy and safety of biologic agents for the treatment of osteoarthritis: a meta-analysis of randomized placebo-controlled trials. Ther Adv Musculoskelet Dis. 2022;14:1–25.

48. Cao Z, Li Y, Wang W, Jie S, Hu X, Zhou J, et al. Is Lutikizumab, an Anti-Interleukin-1alpha/beta Dual Variable Domain Immunoglobulin, efficacious for Osteoarthritis? Results from a bayesian network meta-analysis. Biomed Res Int. 2020;2020:9013283.

49. Cochrane. https://www.cochrane.org (2022). Accessed 20 Aug 2022.

50. Cohen J. Statistical power analysis for the behavioral sciences. Hillsdale: Lawrence Erlbaum Associates; 1988.

51. Fleischmann RM, Bliddal H, Blanco FJ, Schnitzer TJ, Peterfy C, Chen S, et al. A phase II trial of lutikizumab, an anti–interleukin-1α/β dual variable domain immunoglobulin, in knee osteoarthritis patients with synovitis. Arthritis Rheumatol. 2019;71:1056–69.

52. Cohen SB, Proudman S, Kivitz AJ, Burch FX, Donohue JP, Burstein D, et al. A randomized, double-blind study of AMG 108 (a fully human monoclonal antibody to IL-1R1) in patients with osteoarthritis of the knee. Arthritis Res Ther. 2011;13:R125.

53. Baltzer AWA, Moser C, Jansen SA, Krauspe R. Autologous conditioned serum (Orthokine) is an effective treatment for knee osteoarthritis. Osteoarthr Cartil. 2009;17:152–60.

54. Yang KGA, Raijmakers NJH, van Arkel ERA, Caron JJ, Rijk PC, Willems WJ, et al. Autologous interleukin-1 receptor antagonist improves function and symptoms in osteoarthritis when compared to placebo in a prospective randomized controlled trial. Osteoarthr Cartil. 2008;16:498–505.

55. Wang SX, Abramson SB, Attur M, Karsdal MA, Preston RA, Lozada CJ, et al. Safety, tolerability, and pharmacodynamics of an anti-interleukin-1α/β dual variable domain immunoglobulin in patients with osteoarthritis of the knee: a randomized phase 1 study. Osteoarthr Cartil. 2017;25:1952–61.

Yu et al. Journal of Orthopaedic Surgery and Research   (2023) 18:100

Page 16 of 16

56. Chevalier X, Goupille P, Beaulieu AD, Burch FX, Bensen WG, Conrozier T, et al. Intraarticular injection of anakinra in osteoarthritis of the knee: a multicenter, randomized, double-blind, placebo-controlled study. Arthritis Rheum. 2009;61:344–52.

57. Kosloski MP, Goss S, Wang SX, Liu J, Loebbert R, Medema JK, et al. Pharmacokinetics and tolerability of a dual variable domain immunoglobulin ABT-981 Against IL-1α and IL-1β in healthy subjects and patients with osteoarthritis of the knee. J Clin Pharmacol. 2016;56:1582–90.

58. U. S. National Library of Medicine. To determine the safety, tolerability, pharmacokinetics and effect on pain of a single intra-articular administration of canakinumab in patients with osteoarthritis in the knee. https://clinicaltrials.gov/ct2/show/NCT01160822?term=01160822&draw=2&rank=1. Accessed 9 Aug 2022.

59. Brahmachari B, Chatterjee S, Ghosh A. Efficacy and safety of diacerein in early knee osteoarthritis: a randomized placebo-controlled trial. Clin Rheumatol. 2009;28:1193–8.

60. Pelletier JP, Yaron M, Haraoui B, Cohen P, Nahir MA, Choquette D, et al. Efficacy and safety of diacerein in osteoarthritis of the knee: a double-blind, placebo-controlled trial. Arthritis Rheum. 2000;43:2339–48.

61. Pham T, Le Henanff A, Ravaud P, Dieppe P, Paolozzi L, Dougados M. Evaluation of the symptomatic and structural efficacy of a new hyaluronic acid compound, NRD101, in comparison with diacerein and placebo in a 1 year randomised controlled study in symptomatic knee osteoarthritis. Ann Rheum Dis. 2004;63:1611–7.

62. Pavelka K, Trč T, Karpaš K, Viˊtek P, Sedláčková M, Vlasáková Vr, et al. The efficacy and safety of diacerein in the treatment of painful osteoarthritis of the knee: a randomized, multicenter, double-blind, placebo-controlled study with primary end points at two months after the end of a three-month treatment period. Arthritis Rheum. 2007;56:4055–64.

63. van Dalen SCM, Blom AB, Slöetjes AW, Helsen MMA, Roth J, Vogl T, et al. Interleukin-1 is not involved in synovial inflammation and cartilage destruction in collagenase-induced osteoarthritis. Osteoarthr Cartil. 2017;25:385–96.

64. Blumenfeld I, Livne E. The role of transforming growth factor (TGF)-β, insulin-like growth factor (IGF)-1, and interleukin (IL)-1 in osteoarthritis and aging of joints. Exp Gerontol. 1999;34:821–9.

65. Cai H, Sun HJ, Wang YH, Zhang Z. Relationships of common polymorphisms in IL-6, IL-1A, and IL-1B genes with susceptibility to osteoarthritis: a meta-analysis. Clin Rheumatol. 2015;34:1443–53.

66. Chevalier X. Upregulation of enzymatic activity by interleukin-1 in osteoarthritis. Biomed Pharmacother. 1997;51:58–62.

67. Qu Y, Zhou L, Wang C. Mangiferin Inhibits IL-1β-induced inflammatory response by activating PPAR-γ in human osteoarthritis chondrocytes. Inflammation. 2016;40:52–7.

68. Nebbaki SS, El Mansouri FE, Afif H, Kapoor M, Benderdour M, Duval N, et al. Egr-1 contributes to IL-1-mediated down-regulation of peroxisome proliferator-activated receptor γ expression in human osteoarthritic chondrocytes. Arthritis Res Ther. 2012;14:R69.

69. Lin YY, Ko CY, Liu SC, Wang YH, Hsu CJ, Tsai CH, et al. miR-144-3p ameliorates the progression of osteoarthritis by targeting IL-1β: potential therapeutic implications. J Cell Physiol. 2021;236:6988–7000.

70. An Y, Wan G, Tao J, Cui M, Zhou Q, Hou W. Down-regulation of microRNA-203a suppresses IL-1β-induced inflammation and cartilage degradation in human chondrocytes through Smad3 signaling. Biosci Rep. 2020;40:BSR20192723.

71. Lacy SE, Wu C, Ambrosi DJ, Hsieh CM, Bose S, Miller R, et al. Generation and characterization of ABT-981, a dual variable domain immunoglobulin (DVD-Ig(TM)) molecule that specifically and potently neutralizes both IL-1α and IL-1β. MAbs. 2015;7(3):605–19.

72. Arend WP, Malyak M, Guthridge CJ, Gabay C. Interleukin-1 receptor antagonist: role in biology. Annu Rev Immunol. 1998;16:27–55.

73. Sterne JAC, SuttonA J, Ioannidis J, et al. Recommendations for examining and interpreting funnelplot asymmetry in meta-analyses of randomised controlled trials. BMJ. 2011;343:1–8.

Publisher's Note

Springer Nature remains neutral with regard to jurisdictional claims in published maps and institutional affiliations.

Liang *et al. BMC Musculoskeletal Disorders*   (2023) 24:338
https://doi.org/10.1186/s12891-023-06455-1

BMC Musculoskeletal
Disorders

RESEARCH   **Open Access**

Reducing complications of femoral neck fracture management: a retrospective study on the application of multidisciplinary team

Weiming Liang[1†], Gang Qin[1†], Lizhi Yu[1] and Yingying Wang[1*]

Abstract

Background Femoral neck fractures are associated with substantial morbidity and mortality for older adults. Multi-system medical diseases and complications can lead to long-term care needs, functional decline and death, so patients sustaining hip fractures usually have comorbid conditions that may benefit from application of multidisciplinary team(MDT).

Methods This is a retrospective cohort study that incorporates medical record review with an outcomes management database. 199 patients were included who had surgery for a new unilateral femoral neck fracture from January 2018 to December 2021 (96 patients in usual care (UC) model and 103 patients in MDT model. High-energy, pathological, old and periprosthetic femoral neck fracture were excluded. Age, gender, comorbidity status, time to surgery, and postoperative complication, length of stay, in-hospital mortality, 30-day readmission rate, 90-day mortality data were collected and analyzed.

Results Preoperative general data of sex, age, community dwelling and charlson comorbidity score of MDT group (n = 103) have no statistically significant difference with that of usual care (UC) group. Patients treated in the MDT model had significantly shorter times to surgery (38.5 vs. 73.4 h;P = 0.028) and lower lengths of stay (11.5 vs. 15.2 days;P = 0.031). There were no significant differences between two models in In-hospital mortality (1.0% vs. 2.1%; P = 0.273), 30-day readmission rate (7.8% vs. 11.5%; P = 0.352) and 90-day mortality (2.9% vs. 3.1%; P = 0.782). The MDT model had fewer complications overall (16.5% vs. 31.3%; P = 0.039), with significantly lower risks of delirium, postoperative infection, bleeding, cardiac complication, hypoxia, and thromboembolism.

Conclusion Application of MDT can provide standardized protocols and a total quality management approach, leading to fewer complications for elderly patients with femoral neck fracture.

Trial registration No.

Keywords Femoral neck fracture, Multidisciplinary team, Complication

†Weiming Liang and Gang Qin contributed equally to this study.

*Correspondence:
Yingying Wang
WYY15652606080@126.com
[1]The First Affiliated Hospital of Guangxi University of Science and Technology, Guangxi University of Science and Technology, 124 Yuejin Road, Liuzhou 545001, Guangxi Province, China

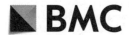

Liang *et al. BMC Musculoskeletal Disorders*   (2023) 24:338

Introduction

Femoral neck fracture is a common injury in orthopedic practice which can cause significant morbidity and mortality [1]. The incidence of femoral neck fractures is increasing due to age-aging reasons, and the risk of fracture doubles every decade after age 50 [2]. Most hip fractures are associated with a fall, although other risk factors include osteoporosis, reduced level of activity, and chronic medication use [3, 4]. The 1-year mortality rate of femoral neck fracture can be up to 30% [5]. Half of the patients were unable to regain pre-fracture mobility, a fourth of whom require long term nursing home care before they had the ability to live independently [6].

Most femoral neck fractures occur in older adults who often have multi-system medical diseases and are at high risk of developing complications such as infection, delirium, and iatrogenic problems [7, 8]. These multi-system medical diseases and complications can lead to long-term care needs, functional decline and death.Surgical decision-making and perioperative management of elderly hip fractures require the joint participation of relevant multidisciplinary physicians including of not only orthopedic surgeons but also doctors of geriatrics, critical care medicine, anesthesiology, mental health department and rehabilitation medicine [9].

Agreed by the international Guidelines, the optimal treatment of hip fractures is immediate surgery for the reduction of the fracture and prosthetic replacement, enhancing the probability of better patient recovery [10]. Arthroplasty (Hemiarthroplasty and total hip replacement) is the treatment of choice for most older individuals who sustain a displaced femoral neck fracture [11]. Long waiting times before intervention will increase complications and mortality for patients with femoral neck fracture [12, 13]. Unfortunately, the surgery was delayed several days after the patient's admission to hospital in many cases, which was seldom attributable to clinical reasons, but was more reasonably due to organizational challenges and bureaucracy [14]. The reasons for the delay could be as follows: patients with femoral neck fracture needed to spend a lot of time queuing for the preoperative examination, because the hospital did not open the preferential pathway for them;doctors of geriatrics waited until the next day to arrive for a consultation;the surgery was postponed due to the chief surgeon's work schedule.

Multidisciplinary team(MDT) is a form of comanagement which has decreased inpatient complications and length of stay [15]. It refers doctors from more than 2 disciplines should conduct consultations for a certain disease, discuss the difficult problems in the diagnosis and treatment of the disease, and finally develop a reasonable and effective treatment plan.

In January 2020, we instituted the MDT program in which elderly patients with femoral neck fractures are admitted to a service comanaged by attending and resident physicians from the internal medicine and orthopaedic surgery departments. We hypothesized that MDT model focused on the care of elderly patients with femoral neck fractures will lead to fewer complications overall compared with usual care (UC).

Methods

Description of MDT and UC models

In UC model, the patient is treated by the orthopedic surgeon after admitted to hospital.The orthopedic surgeon asks the medical history in detail, conducts a systematic and comprehensive evaluation, and adopts general consultation. The relevant examination and treatment should be further implemented according to the consultation opinions. Surgery will be performed after the patient's basic disease is stable and anesthesia consultation opinions is satisfactory.According to the patient's condition after surgery, consultation from other departments will be performed if necessary.Patients with more medical diseases and more severe diseases will be sent to the intensive care unit after surgery. After surgery, the patient's vital signs, mental state, feeding condition, blood routine, biochemical indicators(including of liver function, renal function, myocardial enzyme, electrolyte, blood gas analysis), induced flow rate and cardiopulmonary function were observed, and bilateral limb vascular ultrasound examination was performed. The affected limb was raised, and the quadriceps isolong contraction and ankle pump movement were guided.Prophylactic antibiotics were used within 24 h after surgery.Anticoagulation treatment with rivaroxaban is given routinely. Leaving bed was guided according to fracture type, surgical condition, and systemic condition. Patients with good wound healing, no hip pain, no serious complications, and no serious abnormalities in various laboratory indicators were admitted to discharge.

The MDT team was led by orthopedic surgeons, composed of attending doctors of geriatrics, critical care medicine, anesthesiology, mental health department and rehabilitation medicine. The MDT will evaluate the patient after admission, formulate a personalized examination and treatment plan, open the green channel, shorten the waiting time for examination, adjust the status of the patient to actively prepare for surgery, and shorten the time from admission to operation as far as possible. The surgical treatment plan was identical to the UC group. Patients with more medical diseases and more severe diseases will be sent to the intensive care unit after surgery.Rehabilitation medicine doctors guide the patient to exercise muscle strength and joint mobility, and guide the patient to get early out of bed. Isometric quadriceps

Liang *et al. BMC Musculoskeletal Disorders*　(2023) 24:338

contraction and ankle pump training began 6 h after surgery; knee flexion and straight leg elevation started 1 day after surgery; and walking training with the help of the walker started 2 days after surgery. Other postoperative diagnosis and treatment and discharge criteria were the same as the UC group.

The multidisciplinary team that evaluated the patients was composed of the same people for all patients. All surgeries were performed by the same surgeon.

Study design

This is a retrospective cohort study that incorporates medical record review with an outcomes management database. Information for this database was collected on all patients with femoral neck fractures who complied with the inclusion criteria from January 2018 to December 2021.

Ethical approval and consent

The study was conducted according to the Declaration of Helsinki and the International Conference on Harmonisation Tripartite Guideline on Good Clinical Practice. All patients provided written informed consent before participating. Approvals from Ethics Committee of the First Affiliated Hospital of Guangxi University of Science and Technology were obtained in December 2021(approval number:2021-LC076).

Patients

Inclusion criteria: new unilateral femoral neck fracture patient aged more than or equal to 65 years. Exclusion criteria: fracture due to a high-energy trauma; pathological fractures;old fracture that occurs more than 6 weeks ago; periprosthetic femoral neck fracture. From the electronic database of our hospital, we identified 199 patients who had surgery for a femoral neck fracture from January 2018 to December 2021. Since the initiation of the MDT in January 2020, 96 patients from January 2018 to December 2019 were determined in UC model and 103 patients from January 2020 to December 2021 were determined in MDT model.

Data collected

We collected demographic data, including name, date of birth and gender from the electronic database of our hospital. Inpatient charts (including admission notes, progress notes, operative dictations, consult notes, and discharge summaries) were reviewed to collect the date of admission, date and time of surgery, date of discharge, type of operative repair, comorbid diagnoses and complications. We used Charlson Comorbidity Index [16] to quantify patient comorbidity.

Complications included delirium, postoperative infection, renal insufficiency, bleeding, cardiac, hypoxia,

Table 1 Characteristics of Patients at Baseline

Characteristic	MDT (n = 103)	UC (n = 96)	P value
Age, mean (SD), y	80.6(7.9)	81.2(8.3)	0.631
Male, %	41.2	39.6	0.683
Community dwelling, %	88.3	85.4	0.507
Charlson comorbidity score, mean (SD)	2.2(1.5)	1.9(1.7)	0.131

Table 2 Outcomes in the MDT and UC

Outcome	MDT (n = 103)	UC (n = 96)	P value
Time to surgery, mean (SD), h	38.5(18.6)	73.4(65.8)	0.028
Length of stay, mean (SD), d	11.5(5.6)	15.2(6.8)	0.031
In-hospital mortality, %	1.0	2.1	0.273
30-day readmission rate, %	7.8	11.5	0.352
90-day mortality, %	2.9	3.1	0.782
Complications overall, %	16.5	31.3	0.039
Delirium, %	11.7	23.9	0.032
Postoperative infection, %	7.8	13.5	0.047
Renal insufficiency, %	3.9	5.2	0.092
Bleeding, %	1.0	4.2	0.037
Cardiac, %	1.9	7.3	0.023
Hypoxia, %	3.9	9.4	0.046
Thromboembolism, %	1.0	6.3	0.031
Stroke, %	1.0	2.1	0.241

thromboembolism, stroke. Postoperative infection included urinary tract infection, pneumonia, and surgical site infection. Bleeding included gastrointestinal, retroperitoneal, intracranial bleeding, hemorrhagic stroke, or wound hematoma. Cardiac included any new arrhythmia, acute myocardial infarction, or congestive heart failure.

Statistical analysis

Differences in baseline variables and outcomes between the two models were compared via $\chi2$ analysis for categorical variables, and the Fisher exact test was used for variables with expected cell values less than 5. Continuous variables were compared via the unpaired t test. Differences was considered significant at $P < 0.05$.

Results

Characteristics of the two populations at Baseline are given in Table 1. In the two groups, the comparative differences in preoperative general data of sex, age, community dwelling and charlson comorbidity score were not statistically significant ($P > 0.05$).

The data in Table 2 shows the differences with respect to outcomes between the two models of care. Patients treated in the MDT model had significantly shorter times to surgery (38.5 vs. 73.4 h;P=0.028) and lower lengths of stay (11.5 vs. 15.2 days;P=0.031). There were no significant differences between two models in In-hospital mortality (1.0% vs. 2.1%; P=0.273), 30-day readmission rate (7.8% vs. 11.5%; P=0.352) and 90-day mortality(2.9% vs.

Liang *et al. BMC Musculoskeletal Disorders*   (2023) 24:338

3.1%; P=0.782).The MDT model had fewer complications (16.5% vs. 31.3%; P=0.039), with significantly lower risks of delirium, postoperative infection, bleeding, cardiac complication, hypoxia, and thromboembolism.

Discussion

Our study shows that patients with femoral neck fracture treated in a MDT model of care experience better outcomes than those in the UC model. Specifically, patients in the MDT model underwent surgery approximately one and a half days earlier than those in the UC model. Patients in the MDT model were admitted to discharge approximately four days earlier than those in the UC model.Our study shows substantial promise in decreasing inpatient complications, with MDT patients experiencing a 16.5% complication rate overall vs. 31.3% for UC patients. The complications that were significantly lower in the MDT model were delirium, infection, bleeding,cardiac complications, hypoxia, and thromboembolism. There were no significant differences between two models in In-hospital mortality, 30-day readmission rate and 90-day mortality.

Surgical treatment can avoid the occurrence of bed-related complications in femoral neck fracture patients and reduce the mortality rate [17]. If the patient conditions permit, surgical treatment within 48 h after the injury has become a consensus [11]. Delayed surgery can significantly increase the incidence of complication [12, 13]. However, repeated preoperative consultation and examination of patients will delay the time, and some patients will have various complications while waiting for surgery, losing the timing of surgery [18]. For example, the preoperative chest CT examination indicated that the patient had pneumonia, and then the respiratory department consultation was conducted; after a few days of treatment for pneumonia, the chest CT was reviewed, and then the respiratory department consultation was conducted again; moreover, each consultation or examination might be delayed for one day. Such patients are often complicated with serious medical diseases, and timely and reasonable preoperative evaluation and perioperative management determine the success or failure of the treatment, so it is imperative to implement individualized treatment involving multiple disciplines. The American Society of Anesthesiologists (ASA) classification is strongly associated with medical problems in the perioperative period following hip fracture surgery in the elderly [14]. Patients identified as being at higher risk (in ASA class 3 or 4) preoperatively should be closely managed medically so that perioperative medical complications can be managed and evolving medical issues can be addressed in a timely fashion.

The concept of multidisciplinary team(MDT) was first proposed by the M.D.Anderson Cancer Center in the United States. It refers to discussing the difficult problems in the diagnosis and treatment of patients through consultation in more than two disciplines, and finally formulating a reasonable and effective treatment plan [19]. The concept makes the traditional individual empirical diagnosis and treatment mode into a careful, accurate and reasonable standardized diagnosis and treatment team mode, maximize to avoid the disadvantages of the too fine modern medical branch.It is efficient and convenient, avoid the patients repeated consultation and examination, allow patients enjoy one-stop medical services, and is also an important content of the implementation of postoperative rehabilitation concept.

The purpose of exploring MDT in the treatment of elderly femoral neck fractures is to integrate relevant medical resources, optimize processes, and rationally select treatment plans, so that patients can be treated safely with surgery as soon as possible, and reduce the complication rate and mortality. Recent studies have suggested the management model of MDT results in shorten time to surgery, shorter length of stay, lower complication rates and lower readmission rates [20–22], whose results are similar to ours.The composition of the MDT was similar in previous literature. Loizzo M et al. reported that the collaboration between healthcare system management, orthopedic specialists, geriatric specialist and physical therapists was needed to drive shorter days of hospitalization and better overall patient health outcome by performing surgery as soon as possible [22]. Lau TW et al. reported that their team was composed of not only surgeons, physicians, anaesthetists and nurses, but also the rehabilitation doctors, nurses, therapists and medical social workers in a rehabilitation hospital [9]. In our MDT model, orthopedic surgeons was the leader, and geriatric specialist was responsible for the management of multi-system medical diseases and complications. Anesthesiologist assessed the anesthesia risk and administered anesthesia. Doctors of critical care medicine and mental health department would participate according to the patient's condition.

Advanced age and surgical trauma are well-recognized risk factors for post-operative delirium. Jin et al. retrospectively studied 258 patients with femoral neck fracture data, and found the incidence of postoperative delusion was 17.4% [23]; The mortality rate of patients who develop postoperative delusion is three times as much as the patient without postoperative delusion [24, 25]. In our study, The incidence of postoperative delusion in the MDT group was only 11.7%, which was significantly lower than the 23.9% of patients in the UC group.

Elderly patients with femoral neck fracture have not fully recovered at discharge, and mostly are clinical healing. The functional recovery of patients largely depends on good rehabilitation treatment.In the past, insufficient

Liang *et al. BMC Musculoskeletal Disorders*   (2023) 24:338   Page 5 of 6

attention was paid to the postoperative rehabilitation of such patients, which can lead to artificial joint dislocation, malunion, joint stiffness, deep vein thrombosis and other complications [26]. The MDT model included the rehabilitation physician to provide rehabilitation treatment and guidance to such patients, so that the patients could get out of bed and exercise as soon as possible, and restore the affected limb function to the maximum extent.

In the MDT diagnosis and treatment, the most beneficial group is the high-risk patients with poor systemic condition. Under the cooperation of multidisciplinary doctors, we could implement individualized management in the perioperative period, actively conduct preoperative evaluation, timely and effectively intervene for the combined medical diseases, adjust the functions of patients to the best state for surgical treatment, and finally obtain a good prognosis [20]. Treatment of high-risk femoral neck fracture patients will be difficult to rely on a single discipline. Only by breaking the boundaries of the specialty, with the strength of multidisciplinary comprehensive treatment, and having a comprehensive understanding of the disease, can we provide patients the best treatment plan and improve the doctor-patient relationship, which will also be an inevitable trend of the development of large general hospitals.

There was no significant differences between two models in In-hospital mortality, 30-day readmission rate and 90-day mortality. In this regard, we believe that although patients can benefit from MDT, the extent of the benefit is not yet large enough to affect mortality and 30-day readmission rate.Similar studies also showed that significant differences in mortality cannot be caused by MDT model [15, 26, 27]. It means that MDT models of care may improve short-term outcomes for patients with femoral neck fracture, but it may not yield longer-term benefits. Perhaps long-term prognosis is closely related to the long-term control of multi-system diseases, which is not easily affected by MDT models. More clinical data are needed to confirm this opinion.

Besides, according to our experience, there are many problems that need to be overcome in the specific implementation process. The cognitive differences between disciplines might bring about controversy over treatment options. The cooperation could not operate for a long time due to the lack of performance incentive mechanism. The implementation of MDT needs the support of the hospital management, and a reasonable full top-level design is indispensable.

This study has several limitations. First, our study is a retrospective cohort study which depends on data available from medical record review for identification of comorbidity and complications. These limitations might affect both models and had influence in comparing

outcomes between the two groups.Second, different outcomes between two groups may be attributable to some thing other than the model of care, such as surgical protocols, surgical approach, unmeasured patient characteristics, or nursing care, which were not measured in this study. Our study failed to analyze this information even further. Thir, our medical record review was unblinded, which could have led to bias in determining complications.

In conclusion, care of MDT model can provide standardized protocols and a total quality management approach, leading to fewer complications for elderly patients with femoral neck fracture. Replication of MDT model may improve outcomes for those patients with a common and serious condition. More multi-center, prospective, randomized controlled clinical trials are needed to confirm our results and to improve the management process of MDT.

Abbreviations
MDT   Multidisciplinary team
UC   Usual care

Acknowledgements
Everyone who contributed significantly to this study has been listed.

Author Contribution
W.L. and G.Q. performed the data analyses and wrote the manuscript. W.L. and G.Q. contributed equally to this study. L.Y. helped perform the analysis with constructive discussions. Y.W. is responsible for ensuring that the descriptions are accurate and agreed by all authors. All authors read and approved the final manuscript.

Funding
The authors disclose the receipt of the following financial support for the research, authorship, and/or publication of this article: This work was supported by the Guangxi Natural Science Foundation (AD19245017), the Scientific Research Foundation of Guangxi University of Science and Technology(20Z13), the Scientific Research Foundation of Guangxi Health Commission (Z20211376) and the Scientific Research Foundation of Guangxi Health Commission (Z20190410).

Data Availability
The data that support the findings of this study are available from the corresponding author upon reasonable request.

Declarations

Ethics approval and consent to participate
The study was conducted according to the Declaration of Helsinki and the International Conference on Harmonisation Tripartite Guideline on Good Clinical Practice. All patients provided written informed consent before participating. Approvals from Ethics Committee of the First Affiliated Hospital of Guangxi University of Science and Technology were obtained in December 2021(approval number:2021-LC076).

Consent for publication
Not applicable.

Competing interests
The authors declare that they have no competing interests.

Received: 13 December 2022 / Accepted: 25 April 2023
Published online: 29 April 2023

Liang *et al. BMC Musculoskeletal Disorders*   (2023) 24:338

References

1. Gullberg B, Johnell O, Kanis JA. World-wide projections for hip fracture. Osteoporos Int. 1997;7(5):407–13.
2. Kates SL, Kates OS, Mendelson DA. Advances in the medical management of osteoporosis. Injury. 2007;38(Suppl 3):17–23.
3. LeBlanc KE, Muncie HL Jr, LeBlanc LL. Hip fracture: diagnosis, treatment, and secondary prevention. Am Fam Physician. 2014;15(12):945–51.
4. Scaturro D, Vitagliani F, Terrana P, Tomasello S, Camarda L, Letizia Mauro G. Does the association of therapeutic exercise and supplementation with sucrosomial magnesium improve posture and balance and prevent the risk of new falls? Aging Clin Exp Res. 2022;34(3):545–53.
5. Kristensen PK, Thillemann TM, Søballe K, Johnsen SP. Can improved quality of care explain the success of orthogeriatric units? A population-based cohort study. Age Ageing. 2016;45(1):66–71.
6. Braithwaite RS, Col NF, Wong JB. Estimating hip fracture morbidity, mortality and costs. J Am Geriatr Soc. 2003;51(3):364–70.
7. Inouye SK, Viscoli CM, Horwitz RI, Hurst LD, Tinetti ME. A predictive model for delirium in hospitalized elderly medical patients based on admission characteristics. Ann Intern Med. 1993;119(6):474–81.
8. Creditor MC. Hazards of hospitalization of the elderly. Ann Intern Med. 1993;118(3):219–23.
9. Lau TW, Fang C, Leung F. The effectiveness of a multidisciplinary hip fracture care model in improving the clinical outcome and the average cost of manpower. Osteoporos Int. 2017;28(3):791–8.
10. National Institute for Clinical Excellences. The management of hip fracture in adults. London (UK): NICE clinical guidelines CG124. London: National Institute for Health and Care Excellence, 2011. Available from: http://guidance.nice.org.uk/ CG124 [Last accessed: 2017, Sept 8]. In.
11. Florschutz AV, Langford JR, Haidukewych GJ, Koval KJ. Femoral neck fractures: current management. J Orthop Trauma. 2015;29(3):121–9.
12. Sheehan KJ, Sobolev B, Chudyk A, Stephens T, Guy P. Patient and system factors of mortality after hip fracture: a scoping review. BMC Musculoskelet Disord. 2016;17:166.
13. Vidán MT, Sánchez E, Gracia Y, Marañón E, Vaquero J, Serra JA. Causes and effects of surgical delay in patients with hip fracture: a cohort study. Ann Intern Med. 2011;155(4):226–33.
14. Donegan DJ, Gay AN, Baldwin K, Morales EE, Esterhai JL Jr, Mehta S. Use of medical comorbidities to predict complications after hip fracture surgery in the elderly. J Bone Joint Surg Am. 2010;92(4):807–13.
15. Dy CJ, Dossous PM, Ton QV, Hollenberg JP, Lorich DG, Lane JM. Does a multidisciplinary team decrease complications in male patients with hip fractures? Clin Orthop Relat Res. 2011;469(7):1919–24.
16. Charlson ME, Pompei P, Ales KL, MacKenzie CR. A new method of classifying prognostic comorbidity in longitudinal studies: development and validation. J Chronic Dis. 1987;40(5):373–83.
17. Tay E. Hip fractures in the elderly: operative versus nonoperative management. Singap Med J. 2016;57(4):178–81.
18. Dash SK, Panigrahi R, Palo N, Priyadarshi A, Biswal M. Fragility hip fractures in Elderly Patients in Bhubaneswar, India (2012–2014): a prospective Multicenter Study of 1031 Elderly patients. Geriatr Orthop Surg Rehabil. 2015;6(1):11–5.
19. Collins J, Skilton K. Low vision services in South Devon: a multi-agency, multidisciplinary approach. Ophthalmic Physiol Opt. 2004;24(4):355–9.
20. Gupta A. The effectiveness of geriatrician-led comprehensive hip fracture collaborative care in a new acute hip unit based in a general hospital setting in the UK. J R Coll Physicians Edinb. 2014;44(1):20–6.
21. Leung AH, Lam TP, Cheung WH, Chan T, Sze PC, Lau T, Leung KS. An orthogeriatric collaborative intervention program for fragility fractures: a retrospective cohort study. J Trauma. 2011;71(5):1390–4.
22. Loizzo M, Gallo F, Caruso D. Reducing complications and overall healthcare costs of hip fracture management: a retrospective study on the application of a diagnostic therapeutic pathway in the Cosenza General Hospital. Ann Ig. 2018;30(3):191–9.
23. Jin J, Wang G, Gong M, Zhang H, Liu J. Retrospective comparison of the effects of epidural anesthesia versus peripheral nerve block on postoperative outcomes in elderly chinese patients with femoral neck fractures. Clin Interv Aging. 2015;10:1223–31.
24. Saravay SM, Kaplowitz M, Kurek J, Zeman D, Pollack S, Novik S, Knowlton S, Brendel M, Hoffman L. How do delirium and dementia increase length of stay of elderly general medical inpatients? Psychosomatics 2004, 45(3):235–42.
25. Heyman N, Nili F, Shahory R, Seleznev I, Ben Natan M. Prevalence of delirium in geriatric rehabilitation in Israel and its influence on rehabilitation outcomes in patients with hip fractures. Int J Rehabil Res. 2015;38(3):233–7.
26. Dy CJ, Dossous PM, Ton QV, Hollenberg JP, Lorich DG, Lane JM. The medical orthopaedic trauma service: an innovative multidisciplinary team model that decreases in-hospital complications in patients with hip fractures. J Orthop Trauma. 2012;26(6):379–83.
27. Friedman SM, Mendelson DA, Bingham KW, Kates SL. Impact of a comanaged geriatric fracture Center on short-term hip fracture outcomes. Arch Intern Med. 2009;169(18):1712–7.

Publisher's Note

Springer Nature remains neutral with regard to jurisdictional claims in published maps and institutional affiliations.